Emerging Values in Health Care

of related interest

The Challenge of Practical Theology
Selected Essays
Stephen Pattison
ISBN 978 1 84310 453 7

Living with Learning Disabilities, Dying with Cancer
Thirteen Personal Stories
Irene Tuffrey-Wijne
Foreword by Sheila Hollins
ISBN 978 1 84905 027 2

Betraying the NHS
Health Abandoned
Michael Mandelstam
ISBN 978 1 84310 482 7

Partnerships in Social Care
A Handbook for Developing Effective Services
Keith Fletcher
ISBN 978 1 84310 380 6

Emerging Values
in Health Care
The Challenge for Professionals

Edited by Stephen Pattison, Ben Hannigan,
Roisin Pill and Huw Thomas

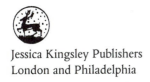

Jessica Kingsley Publishers
London and Philadelphia

First published in 2010
by Jessica Kingsley Publishers
116 Pentonville Road
London N1 9JB, UK
and
400 Market Street, Suite 400
Philadelphia, PA 19106, USA

www.jkp.com

Library of Congress Cataloging in Publication Data

A CIP catalog record for this book is available from the Library of Congress

British Library Cataloguing in Publication Data

A CIP catalogue record for this book is available from the British Library

ISBN 978 1 84310 947 1

Printed and bound in Great Britain by
MPG Books Limited

This book is for

KIERAN SWEENEY

with thanks for all he has contributed to the
theory and practice of health care

from some of the colleagues who have been
fortunate enough to work with him

Contents

Preface

This book is the fruit of a four-year conversation about professional values in health care. The dialogue has been conducted by a small interdisciplinary and interprofessional group of nurses, doctors, pharmacists, clergy, planners, sociologists, linguists, psychologists, philosophers and theologians, based mainly at Cardiff University. While we have never got around formally to designating ourselves 'The Cardiff Professional Values Group', that is how we think of ourselves.

In 2004, the group, then in its infancy with only three years of mutual exploration behind it, published a more general volume, *Values in Professional Practice* (edited by Stephen Pattison and Roisin Pill). While there was a good deal about health professionals in that general volume, the present volume focuses particularly on health professionals and their changing roles, values and contexts mainly within the British National Health Service (NHS). It is the examination of changes in values – as espoused and/or as practised – which distinguishes this book from our earlier one. All the members of the group have written chapters in the present volume – and you can meet them in their writing and in their short biographies.

On this occasion, we are also lucky to have a number of critical interlocutors, chosen because of their rootedness in professional work in current health care practice, who have written responses to the majority of the main chapters. We are very grateful to these individuals for giving up their very precious time to write with us, and thank them for their care in producing responses that should greatly enrich the dialogue about values and health care practice for readers.

The authors and respondents were fortunate to be invited to share their drafts and ideas together at a day seminar sponsored by the Nuffield Trust and held at its London headquarters in July 2008. We acknowledge with gratitude the encouragement and support given to the group by Nuffield on this and other occasions. In this connection we should mention the particular support of Dame Carol Black and Jennifer Dixon, respectively chair and chief executive of Nuffield, and the wonderful practical facilitation of the seminar provided by Kerry Jones and Kate Uvelli Howe. We were also fortunate enough to have with us a number of guests who enriched our discussions with their perceptive insights: David Armstrong (King's College London), Alistair Hewison (University of Birmingham), Ian Hulatt (Royal College of Nursing) and Albert Weale (University of Essex). Many thanks are due to each of them, as they are also to Jessica Kingsley and her colleagues at the eponymous publishing house who have worked so hard and well to get the contents of this book out of our heads and into readers' hands.

The editors would also like formally to thank chapter authors and respondents for their prompt cooperation in producing and amending drafts to meet a number of stiff deadlines.

We hope that readers will gain from the pages that follow a clear sense of the interest and importance of interprofessional and interdisciplinary discussion about values in professions involved in the NHS. Values are not the province of any particular group of theorists or practitioners. Thus, a multi-vocal, multi-faceted approach to health care professions and professionals seems highly appropriate. Would that there was more critical discussion of values within and between health care professions, and with the users they serve. If this book helps to stimulate such dialogue, the labours of all who have contributed to this book will not have been in vain.

Stephen Pattison
Ben Hannigan
Roisin Pill
Huw Thomas
July 2009

Introduction

Stephen Pattison and Huw Thomas

Values talk is everywhere in contemporary Britain. While politicians laud the importance of developing specifically British values that all citizens can affirm, businesses claim to be value-led and firms that wish to enhance their attractiveness emphasize the importance of their values. However, 'values' remain profoundly slippery, carrying different meanings for different people in different contexts.[1] This slipperiness has not stopped talk of values becoming increasingly prominent and important in public service institutions over the last two decades, including in the National Health Service (NHS).

Often it is the NHS, perhaps more than other public bodies, which is taken to embody the fundamental, decent values and aspirations of British society. It may be surprising, then, that it was not until 2009 that the NHS in England articulated for itself a formal set of values within its new Constitution (Department of Health 2009). But this curious omission does not mean that articulate values discourse and usage has been absent within the NHS: professions and other groups have been formulating and re-formulating their values and principles by way of codes and other documents with increasing frequency for a long time now.

The context of the increasing attention to overtly expressed values and values talk is that of continuing change. Arguably, when society and social groups are fairly static and calm everyone implicitly understands how things work and what particular occupations do; there is no need

---

[1] For background to discussion about the nature of values and professions generally, see Pattison and Pill (2004). There, contributions explore (amongst other areas) the nature and pluriform meanings of the concept of 'values', and the differences between values that are espoused and those which are enacted. For a broad background to NHS values in particular see New and Neuberger (2002).

to attend explicitly to values. It is only when norms and customs are problematized, institutions change their structures and functions, professional roles change and blur, and individuals are required to become ever more flexible, that it becomes necessary to articulate identities, boundaries and functions. And it is at times like these that overt values talk comes to the fore.

There can be no doubt that the NHS has seen an enormous amount of change at all levels in the past couple of decades. Several fundamental structural revolutions have occurred. New occupational groups have emerged, while some old ones have disappeared or been subsumed into others. Some professions have become more numerous and stronger, gaining a clearer sense of identity and purpose. Others have changed direction. While at the inception of the NHS in 1948 health care was institutionally based, much health care is now based in the community and delivered by a great variety of medical and paramedical groups. Purchasers and providers of care decreasingly see themselves as parts of the same organization, and some providers of services are no longer state owned or run. The NHS in the four devolved countries of the UK is now increasingly developing different identities and practices (see Greer and Rowland 2007). Within this overall flux and change, professionals are becoming more specialized, but are also being required to be more flexible, so that institutional occupational roles may no longer be coterminous with professional boundaries and skills. The chief executive of a health care service or trust may be a doctor, a nurse or an occupational therapist, or may have no clinical background at all. A prescriber may be a doctor, a nurse or a pharmacist. Increasingly, health care professionals are being encouraged or required to view themselves as part of a multi-disciplinary team.

Given the plurality, diversity and fragmentation of contexts, institutions, groups and roles, then, it is perhaps to be expected that organizations, professional groups and individuals will want to invest more time in thinking about their own distinctive purposes, roles and identities. And this process of definition and negotiation of boundaries is partly achieved through the language of values. It is when the NHS is threatening to fragment and become pluriform and localized that an attempt is made to formulate national values that continue to give it a sense of unity and distinctive identity. It is almost as if the expression of values is an exercise in nostalgia, trying to put back in place a (possibly imaginary) united sense of purpose, meaning and identity that might, in fact, already have been lost.

This book analyses some of the changes that have taken place in values usage and talk as organizations, professions and professionals have found themselves immersed in rapid and fundamental change. If organizational structures and values change, this affects the context in which professional values are formulated and enacted. Furthermore, as professions change to meet new contexts and challenges while maintaining identity, meaning and purpose, they change the contexts and other professional groups with which they work. It will be seen in the essays that follow that there are many different kinds of values, both espoused and enacted, within professional work in the health care sphere. These values differ enormously in their nature and significance, both within and between professions. Furthermore, at different sites and different levels of health care work and organization, values may serve different functions and play out very differently in their operationalization. Not all professional values are internally consistent and understood, nor are they acted upon in the same way by members of particular professional groups – but, then, the values of different professions may not always be commensurable with those of other groups, or indeed, with those of health care organizations and the NHS as a whole.

What, then, are values, and why might they exercise professionals in a changing health service? Values can be thought of as integral to frameworks for understanding the world and guiding behaviour, attitudes and actions in it. They help us understand the world, and it should be no surprise that the rapidity and radical nature of change in the NHS has induced reflection by professionals on the frameworks within which sense can be made of the changes and their worth.

There are also some more specific functions that values can perform, which may go some way to explaining why value-talk has become so widespread in health care professions:

- *Values legitimize action and organizational arrangements.* An example of this is the way that professional autonomy has historically been justified, at least in part, by the claim that professions use their expertise to pursue socially valued ends altruistically.

- *Values help coordinate action.* There are many ways in which actions of individuals and institutions can be coordinated, but there can be no doubt that coordination can be easier if there are shared values between actors, simply because priorities can then be discussed in instrumental rather than the more intractable moral-political terms. Thus the newly minted NHS Constitution (in England, 2009) can be interpreted in part as an attempt to define a base on which coordinated action between professions, tiers and other interests in this complex body can be improved.

- *Values can be used to discipline/help manage people.* If individuals and groups can be persuaded to adopt certain values, they may be more likely to act in accordance with them than if they ignored such values entirely. There are important qualifications to be made to this, of course. Behaviour (and values) can be shaped by a wide range of factors in an individual's (or group's) day-to-day experience of work, or life more generally. Yet, in codes of ethics, and – arguably – in the managerial vocabulary of outputs, outcomes and efficiency, it is possible to perceive attempts to get individuals to internalize values that will be functional for the organizational unit of which they are a part.

- *Values justify change – and resistance to change.* Attempts to alter the nature or trajectory of an organization radically are often justified, and resisted, by reference to values that will be promoted (or damaged) thereby.

- *Values help create and consolidate identity.* Hence values are often central to boundary maintenance between professions. On the whole, values are not easily changed or supplanted, because doing so entails a significant change in personal or group identity. The attention that is sometimes paid to tracing continuity of values between historically significant figures in a profession and contemporary practitioners can perhaps be explained in part as an attempt to establish the contemporary professional as the legitimate heir of the revered forebear – i.e. to support the claim that the profession's identity has remained, in certain key respects, unchanged.

It can be argued that values, particularly of the idealistic, aspirational and ethical kind, are not very influential in health care policy – following the cart of pragmatism rather than leading the way (Klein 2007). But whether or not values are fundamental or somewhat epi-phenomenal, much effort is put into identifying and agreeing upon their nature. It seems likely, then, that the formulation and discussion of values is in some way fundamental to maintaining and enhancing organizational and professional identities. If this is so, it is important to understand the nature, usage and context of professional values in health care.

In confusing times of change and uncertainty, professions, professionals, their clients and their employers need to be able to articulate and examine their own values. They also need to be able to understand the values of others. If the value of patient-centred, seamless care (a popular value in many professions and organizations) is to be realized, for example, it is important to understand how competing and compatible values in different professional groups might inhibit or foster collaboration. Teamwork and trust (two other important values in specialized, highly specialized and differentiated health work) may remain effectively impossible if professionals, individually and collectively, fail to understand and appreciate the value stances and identities of other groups. So assaying something of the nature and importance of espoused and enacted values is a vital practical task in the contemporary NHS for all those who work in, and use, it. And appreciating the ways in which all values are constantly being renegotiated, re-interpreted and changed as both professions and their contexts evolve is vital if one is to have a realistic view of the possibilities and constraints that surround health care provision and work.

WHAT THIS BOOK DOES

In order to better understand the changing nature and significance of values and how they intersect with professional practice in particular contexts, the essays in this book probe selectively into the life and work of several professions at different levels and in different ways. The book does not attempt to be comprehensive or consistently to apply methods or approaches to the changing nature of values and professions. Rather, it invites readers to read different professions, different values and different contexts through a diverse range of lenses that reflect the interests, backgrounds and skills of the authorial team. In itself, this bears witness to the diversity of methods and approaches that can be taken to the diverse field of professions and values. Values, professions or organizations are not unitary phenomena that can and should be approached always in the same way. This book, therefore, honours the complexity of not just the overall picture of how living values interact with professional practices and contexts, but also the possible methods and approaches that might be used to understand them.

The authors of the chapters herewith have worked as an interdisciplinary, interprofessional team to create this volume. Some of us are insiders in the professions about which we write (a couple of us are nurses, a couple have backgrounds in management); others are long-term observers of particular professions and their development, or are engaged in actively training professionals. One or two of us are academic theorists with philosophical analytical skills.

These different backgrounds are reflected to some extent in the approaches we have taken to particular values and professions. Some authors (Monrouxe and Sweeney, Chapter 3; Pattison and McKeown, Chapter 10; Sarangi, Chapter 8) approach the subject of changing values through empirical case study analysis or interviews with contemporary professionals. In some other contributions (Hannigan, Chapter 5; Pill, Chapter 4) a documentary, literary, sociological or historical approach is used. Some authors are mainly descriptive in their approach to professions and values, while there are some who are more critical or normative. The nature of the data used varies from documents to interviews. An organizational, political or structural contextual approach to professions and changing professional values is to be found in some chapters (Edgar, Chapter 2), while others are intimately concerned with the development of individual professionals and their identities and value manipulation in everyday life (Badcott, Chapter 7). Some of the professions studied here are well established, dominant and well known to the public (general practitioners, general nurses), while others are more marginal or minority groups (genetic counsellors, chaplains), more recently established (mental health nurses), or still trying to establish their significance (pharmacists). For some professional groups, like mental health nurses, values are central to their quest for recognition. For others, values are less overtly important; medicine, for example, has probably never doubted that it is informed by excellent values, even if it would not characterize itself as 'value-led'. Whatever the profession, level or approach, all these groups are fundamentally influenced by organizational, political and social context.

The first two chapters provide background and context for the later chapters, which can be seen as case studies of aspects of value evolution and usage in different professional groups. In the first chapter, the authors trace the origins of some significant professional groups and practices in the UK, as well as providing a clear picture of the professional composition and numbers of people working in particular NHS occupations today. This chapter reveals the diverse, pluralistic and changing nature of health care professions and some of the challenges they face. This picture is adumbrated and amplified in Chapter 2, where Andrew Edgar, a philosopher, sketches in the socio-political forces that bear in upon professions and professional work in the NHS today. Again, Edgar sketches out the historical background to the evolution of health care organization and practice. This has a crucial influence on the nature of professional values and practice, making it clear that the State has a major role in determining values and practice in health care.

Chapters 3 to 10 examine aspects of changing values in individual professions. In each case, the chapter is followed by a response from a reflective practitioner, providing readers with a second perspective on many of the key matters discussed.

It is doctors who are the focus of attention in Chapters 3 and 4. Chapter 3 starts with the formation of individual professionals in medical education. Lynn Monrouxe and Kieran Sweeney, themselves medical educators as well as trained practitioners, use a detailed case study of one episode in the training of a doctor to trace the ways in which subtle adjustments are made in an attempt to establish congruence between personal and enacted professional values. The chapter may prompt questions about the extent to which a tension between personal and professional/organizational values may not be a bad thing in an imperfect world: how easily should we sleep? (This is a question that Sellman's discussion of adult general nursing (see Chapter 6) might also help to address.) It is the power relations embedded in the episode under discussion that most strike respondent Brian Hurwitz. In his response he suggests that social relations are power-laden as well as value-laden. Thus, the thinking through of values in professional life cannot be divorced from thinking about appropriate relations of power.

In Chapter 4, Roisin Pill, a medical sociologist, reviews the evidence available about the changing nature of general practice. The chapter's historical perspective reminds us that the NHS has always been an organization subject to change. Yet there can be little doubt that as far as general practice is concerned particularly far-reaching change appears to be currently under way. She delineates a professional group that may well be in the process of fragmentation, with value-laden notions such as vocation appearing to be increasingly irrelevant to some emerging forms of general practice. While Pill implies that many general practitioners are broadly supportive of the changes under way (in that they are choosing career trajectories that suit their personal aspirations), her respondent, Paquita de Zulueta, is less sanguine. She sketches a picture of a profession under pressure to uphold core values in an increasingly unsupportive bureaucratic and commercialized context.

What might be the appropriate relationship between professional and 'patient'/service user is something that mental health nursing has wrestled with over the past 40 years. Ben Hannigan's historical account, in Chapter 5, of a relatively recently professionalized occupation provides something of a contrast to many others in the book, which emphasize dilemmas and crises facing health care professions. Hannigan reviews the way in which major policy documents have conceptualized the nature of mental health nursing, and the role of values within it – which is an important one since the profession overtly considers itself as 'value-led'. One interesting strand he identifies is the way in which the working practices of researching and developing the policy documents have changed in step with changes in the statements' characterization of mental health nursing. A rather inward-looking, medicalized approach to understanding nursing has been replaced by an openness to a wider array of perspectives on what is done and what constitutes success. While aware of the limitations of largely documentary evidence, both Hannigan and Bronwen Davies, his respondent, think that in certain respects mental health nursing is in a better state today than it was decades ago. Central to the progress made has been the explicit acknowledgement within the values promoted by the professionalizing occupation of mental health nursing of the humanity and dignity of the users of mental health services. As with any health care profession, changes such as these emerge from a complex interaction of governmental, professional and pressure group activity. In the case of mental health nursing, service users appear to be better respected by professionals, though the service as a whole remains a Cinderella within the NHS – perhaps the more so because its value base increasingly takes it away from the values supporting a biomedical model of treatment (see Chapter 1).

Derek Sellman's focus, in Chapter 6, is on a different kind of nursing, adult general nursing – the kind we encounter when we have an accident, or enter hospital to have our appendix removed. Sellman's philosophical reflection builds on the work of Alasdair MacIntyre, to establish that there will be an inevitable tension between values that define what it is to do nursing properly and excellently, and the requirements of the institutional infrastructure that makes nursing provision possible in a modern, mass society. Inevitable as a degree of tension may be, it is still important to sound a warning bell when institutional demands threaten core values of the practice of nursing – when they begin to undermine the very thing that the institution is there to enable. Both Sellman and his respondent Christine Hockley fear that this is the position today in the NHS. Organizational models, they suggest, as well as the associated values imported into the NHS, undermine the very practice of nursing. Yet Christine Hockley's contribution also illustrates the significance of human agency, and local responses. The NHS is not monolithic: individual units at a very small scale may devise approaches that go some way to safeguarding important intrinsic values. What allows for this room for manœuvre, how it is exploited, and the skills needed to do so, are themselves interesting topics for empirical research.

Pharmacy and adult general nursing are very different kinds of occupations, but they share dilemmas arising from the potential of institutional context to undermine, or otherwise bring into question, fundamental values. David Badcott's account of pharmacy (Chapter 7) shows how its straddling of two rather different institutional contexts – the bureaucracy of the NHS (notably in hospitals) and the market – imposes peculiar strains. A (curiously belated) code of ethics may be simply a standard marker of professionalism in the NHS. However, it is clear from what Badcott and his respondent Alan Nathan say that this imposes demands that pharmacists in the private sector (especially if employees of large firms) find difficult to meet. The development of the code of ethics appears to be an illustration of values-talk being used as part of a wider strategy of boundary-marking in a fluid organizational context. Hospital chaplains are responding to these pressures, too (see Chapter 9).

Most of the discussions in this book concern professions in which there appears to be a fair amount of agreement among professionals themselves about the fundamental nature and purpose of their activity. Even in the case of general practice, where a number of models of service delivery are now emerging, there is no suggestion of significant debate about fundamental purpose and values. Perhaps it is the relative newness of genetic counselling (the professionalizing occupation that Srikant Sarangi discusses in Chapter 8) that explains the lively discussions he reviews (and to which his respondent, Heather Skirton, contributes) about the core purpose of counselling. Using discourse analyses of episodes in genetic counselling, Sarangi explores the complex, sometimes confused, interplay of different approaches to counselling – each with their different value-bases. Counsellors and users of their services grapple with problems in which it is evidently difficult to keep apart personal and professional values and orientations (see also Chapter 3 on medical education). Heather Skirton is convinced of the need to do so, but Derek Sellman's approach to professional values would imply a great degree of congruence between personal and professional life, a congruence implied by the term 'vocation'.

The analysis presented of hospital chaplaincy by Paul Ballard in Chapter 9 poses serious questions about where vocation as traditionally understood might fit into the emerging model of chaplaincy in the NHS. His respondent, Chris Swift, is surely right to be wary of the way in which vocation has been used to justify the exploitation of health care workers, but there can be no doubt that this notion is also central to the relationship of personal and professional life and values. Chaplains appear to be intent on professionalizing in a form that is bureaucratically appropriate for the NHS. They want to be part of the health care team. Ballard explains what that means in a body managed by principles of the new public management (see Chapter 1) and necessarily sensitive to its increasingly non-Christian users. The changes under way raise questions about why a chaplain needs any religious faith at all. And it is fascinating that a professional group that might be thought historically to provide both a repository of values and skills is, in addressing and implementing them, caught up in the flux and uncertainty of values discussion in the NHS.

There may be ambiguity about the role of faith and values in the work of NHS chaplains, but NHS hospital managers have been characterized as among those propagating a new faith – that of management theory, which is inimical to many of the values for which health care workers believe they stand. However, the literature review and empirical study of a sample of managers reported by Pattison and McKeown in Chapter 10 shows that often managers espouse values that are central to a rather conventional, time-honoured view of the NHS. While NHS managers may have an eye to the bottom line and the needs of all rather than of particular individuals in a clinical setting, they are curiously very committed to the founding values of the NHS and public service. Perhaps this is sometimes belied in practice, but it is interesting to see stereotypes of managers as vectors of values such as economy and efficiency without care for the public or individual good being challenged. Moira Dumma, in her response to the article, expresses some scepticism about the accuracy of this stereotype in any case. She argues that even if it has some truth in it, new mechanisms such as the values embodied in the NHS Constitution will act to focus and unite clinicians and managers in a common purpose driven essentially by values centred on patient care and social wellbeing – so there is no scope for demonizing managers in the values debate.

There are a number of themes that emerge from many of the chapters in the book. Among the more prominent are these:

- Values are profoundly implicated in identity-formation and boundary-marking between professions.

- There are important and sometimes painful tensions between institutional forms and professional values and practices.

- Work is required in order to reconcile tensions between personal and professional values (and there are questions about the desirability of such reconciliation).

- Power-relations are significant in values talk, formulation and implementation between all those in the NHS (including users). Values are implicated in both legitimizing and questioning such relations.

- Different professionalized occupations have very different historical trajectories and intersections with values.

These are among the matters that need serious and sustained attention from all those with an interest in the NHS. We will return to them, along with other concerns, in a final chapter in which we trace out issues and directions for futher exploration.

REFERENCES

Department of Health (2009) *The NHS Constitution*. London: Department of Health.

Greer, S. and Rowland, D. (eds) (2007) *Devolving Policy, Diverging Values: The Values of the United Kingdom's National Health Services*. London: The Nuffield Trust.

Klein, R. (2007) 'Values Talk in the (English) NHS.' In S. Greer and D. Rowland (eds) *Devolving Policy, Diverging Values: The Values of the United Kingdom's National Health Services*. London: The Nuffield Trust.

New, B. and Neuberger, J. (eds) (2002) *Hidden Assets: Values and Decision-making in the NHS*. London: King's Fund.

Pattison, S. and Pill, R. (eds) (2004) *Values in Professional Practice: Lessons for Health, Social Care and Other Professions*. Oxford: Radcliffe.

Chapter 1

Changing Health Care, Changing Professions

Roisin Pill and Ben Hannigan

INTRODUCTION

We provide here a brief overview of recent developments in the delivery of health care in the UK leading up to the present day, and consider the emergence of (and challenges to) some of the occupational groups found in this field. As a medical sociologist and a nurse, respectively, we bring our own particular disciplinary perspectives to bear; this affects what we choose to include and emphasize here. We are aware, too, that – as noted in this book's Introduction – we are trading in slippery concepts. The idea of the 'professional', and notions such as 'professionalization', are potentially fraught and no consensus exists on their precise meaning (see Pill *et al.* 2004). Our aim, then, is simply to provide a framework for those readers who may not be particularly familiar with the sequencing of events in the history of the National Health Service (NHS), and also to introduce some of the concepts and theories that have been employed in describing, analysing and debating the implications of the major changes which have taken place over this period.

The interdisciplinary group responsible for initiating this book started from the premise that values, particularly those held by men and women providing healing and/or care for the sick and vulnerable, are important subjects to study and debate. They are important because they underpin the way in which care is actually delivered, the nature of the interaction between the carer (who may or may not be a health professional) and the sick person. As Stacey (1988, p.5) points out, 'health work is people work'; moreover, historically such work was largely unpaid and carried out by women, most often mothers, wives and daughters. It will be apparent that such unwaged health care continues to play an important role today – and, indeed, official policy has often relied heavily on these workers for its implementation. Here, however, we are focusing on health occupations in modern Britain: those who are paid for their work in a narrowly defined health care sector in an industrial society with a highly developed division of labour. First, however, there is a brief account of changes in the delivery of health care in the UK since the establishment of the National Health Service in 1948, in order to establish the context in which health professionals have been, and are, working.

THE NATIONAL HEALTH SERVICE FROM 1948[1]
The early years
The establishment of the NHS after World War II by a Labour government has naturally received a great deal of attention from historians, sociologists, health professionals and politicians – all of whom have their own particular perspectives on its antecedents and implications. What cannot be doubted is its importance and its consequences, both intended and unintended. What is also very striking about the planning for this reform is, first, the important role played by the medical profession and, second, those who were *not* included in the discussions. As Klein (1983, p.9) has put it: 'The majority of those actually working in the health services: from nurses to floor sweepers' were excluded. Nor was there formal representation for patients, i.e. those later to be considered as 'consumers'. These arrangements thus strongly reflected the hierarchical and male-dominated nature of British society at that time.

The radical – and enduring – feature of the new NHS was that health care was to be free at the point of delivery to everyone in Britain. Then, as now, the main source of funds was to be general taxation; the health component of the insurance stamp was simply a token. Private treatment remained available for those with money who wished to buy it, but they still had to pay their tax and insurance contributions to the state health

---

1   The start of the NHS is an arbitrary starting point for an exploration of health care in the
    UK, though justified both by its crucial importance in this country's history and reasons of
    space. Those readers interested in the history of healing practices and health care, and the
    development of the professions of medicine and nursing pre-NHS, are referred to the following:
    Albrecht, Fitzpatrick and Scrimshaw 2000; Dingwall, Rafferty and Webster 1998; Porter 1996,
    1997; Stacey 1988.

service. The local authorities lost their hospitals but retained preventive and public health, maternity and infant welfare, and school health. The nationalized hospitals were to be run by appointed boards upon which the local authorities had some seats. The NHS was now the largest British industry and therefore the largest employer. But, of all the health occupations, doctors alone were involved in its management.

Subsequent key changes in the structure of the NHS

THE 1970 REFORMS

Over the following decades it became clear that universally available health care did not in fact, as had been assumed, result in the improvement of the health of the nation, and the rapidly rising cost of the service aroused growing anxiety in governments and therefore also ministry officials. The perceived need for greater control over the activities of doctors and reform of the administrative structure were debated in the 1960s and culminated in the reforms of 1974, which created a three-tier service administered at regional, area and district level. The intention was to produce an integrated service, by unifying the three arms of the NHS: public health, hospital services and general practice. There was also to be responsibility upwards to managerial authority. However, doctors as a whole succeeded in retaining 'clinical autonomy', so that they could be fully responsible for the treatment they prescribed for patients – thus removing themselves from the managerial authority to which all other health care workers were now to be subject. In these ways the medical profession managed to limit the aims of integration and managerialism (Allsop 1984; Levitt 1979).

THE CONSERVATIVES, GENERAL MANAGEMENT AND THE MARKET

A turning point in the history of welfare came in 1979 with the election of a mould-breaking government under the leadership of Margaret Thatcher. Among the Conservatives' first concerns were controlling public spending and improving services through the importation and use of private sector ideas. This government was also willing (unlike previous administrations, but not unlike its New Labour successors) to challenge professional power directly. Managerialism arrived in the NHS with the delivery of Roy Griffiths' brief report to government in 1983, which urged rapid change (Griffiths 1983). Mrs Thatcher's government was swift to act on Griffiths' recommendations, and by the middle of the 1980s was directing local NHS organizations to begin the task of appointing general managers (Powell 2000). Other features of what Hood (1991) has since called the 'new public management' followed. Doctors were encouraged to accept responsibility for the resource implications of their clinical decision-making. Whilst reaffirming that the NHS should continue to be funded through general taxation, the White Paper *Working for Patients* (Department of Health 1989) aroused immediate health professional resistance by proposing the introduction of market mechanisms. Many working in the health service feared that competition would undermine the principles of equity and access for all (Ham 1996).

Opposition notwithstanding, at the start of the following decade *Working for Patients* became incorporated into the NHS and Community Care Act (1990), a piece of legislation significant for at least three reasons (Klein 1998):

- The introduction of an internal market meant that district health authorities were handed the responsibility to purchase services based on their assessments of local health need, and newly formed NHS trusts were given the task of providing services.

- GPs were granted the opportunity to become independent fundholders, and to purchase care and treatment using budgets devolved to the level of local practices.

- The Act reinforced the requirement to promote health care quality, efficiency and effectiveness.

Research evidence into the impact of the internal market is sparse (Le Grand 1999). Le Grand observes, however, that at the very least the purchaser/provider reforms of the 1990s exerted a lasting influence on NHS culture and ways of working. By granting new power to general practitioners (GPs) through the introduction of fundholding, for example, the balance of power tilted away from hospitals and their consultants towards family doctors. This largely remains the case today. The move towards the use of market mechanisms, and its associated emphases on effectiveness and efficiency, has also endured, and has proved of lasting consequence for the work and position of professionals.

NEW LABOUR, MODERNIZATION AND PATIENTS' RIGHTS

Ahead of its landslide victory in 1997 New Labour campaigned for a 'Third Way' for the UK's public services, and, once elected, acted swiftly to initiate a programme of 'modernization'. However, despite New Labour's rhetoric on undoing the internal market reforms of previous administrations, in significant respects the new government's earliest plans for change represented an extension of what had gone before, rather than a revolution (Klein 1998; Le Grand 1999). The separation of purchasing from providing was to remain, albeit with a new requirement for organizations to collaborate rather than compete. Fundholding was to be abolished, but primary care was to retain its position at the centre of local commissioning. Care-providing NHS trusts were to be retained. In addition, no new money was – at first – to be made available for the development of services, with extra resources planned to come from cost savings associated with reductions in bureaucracy.

Early New Labour action in the health care arena did herald some departures, however. Improving health, in addition to treating illness, was an important new component of the government's programme (Evans 2004). With an emphasis on improving quality in health care, early initiatives also included the introduction of a new framework for local service improvement – 'clinical governance' – and the launching of two new bodies: the Commission for Health Improvement (CHI, which via subsequent reorganizations and changes in remit has now become, in England, the Care Quality Commission) and the National Institute for Clinical Excellence (NICE, now known in England and Wales as the National Institute for Health and Clinical Excellence). The former was responsible for assessing the quality of provision through routine reviews of NHS organizations, and by conducting one-off investigations where concerns over poor standards existed. The latter was to produce guidance for professionals and the public on the provision of effective treatments. In another significant departure from the wider policies pursued by its predecessor, New Labour also acted on its commitment to devolution. By facilitating the creation of separate administrations in Scotland and Wales in its first term of office, the government created conditions favourable for the development of marked differences in the future shape of the health service across the territories of the UK.

New Labour set about its early public services modernization programme at a frenetic pace (6 and Peck 2004), and to a large degree the scale and speed of change since the middle of the 1990s has continued.

Plans to raise the proportion of the UK's gross domestic product devoted to health care to nearer the European average were announced in 2000 (Dixon 2001). In the same year an ambitious long-term strategy, badged as a partnership between government and the professions, was launched with the aim of improving the health of the population of England (Department of Health 2000). Similar strategies appeared elsewhere in the UK. Along with the promise of extra resources in the form of more doctors, nurses and other professionals came demands for closer scrutiny of performance and greater accountability (Greener 2004).

HEALTH PROFESSIONALS IN THE NHS

It is apparent that the context for professional practice in the NHS has changed significantly in the past ten or so years, but so has the character and composition of the workforce. The NHS is still, by far, the major provider of health care in the UK. All the training received by doctors and nurses is provided by the public sector and nearly all trained health professionals work in the public sector (Buchan 2006). Staff work in a variety of organizations in primary or community care (where, usually, the first point of contact for patients is via their local GP) or in secondary care (usually hospitals) where specialized treatment is given.

Given the size and complexity of the health service and its constituent organizations, generating accurate and up-to-date information on the workforce is something of a challenge. At the time of writing the most recent data is available from 2004 (Department of Health 2005). At that time approximately 1.3 million people were employed in the NHS, on a head-count basis, representing an average increase of over 39,000 per year since 1997. This number included 660,706 professionally qualified clinical staff, of whom 117,036 were doctors and 397,515 nurses, midwives or health visitors. Qualified scientific, therapeutic and technical staff (ST&T) (including members of the allied health professions, such as occupational therapists, clinical psychologists, radiographers, dieticians, and so on) numbered 128,883, and 17,272 were qualified ambulance workers. A further 368,285 staff worked in clinical support roles in three key areas (support to doctors and nurses, to ST&T staff and to ambulance staff). Running the modern health service also requires large numbers of people to work in infrastructure support roles, and in 2004 a total of 211,489 staff (including 37,726 managers and senior managers) were employed in this category. General practice staff, excluding practice nurses (separately counted in numbers of total nurses), numbered 90,110.

The sheer size of the qualified workforce and its growth (when the data reproduced above were gathered, further staff increases were planned to 2006) reflect the current complexity of the health care sector arising from advances in medical knowledge, the ever-growing importance of technology and the changing needs of a population that is now not only living longer but likely to have more than one chronic condition. Behind the bare figures lies a story of increasing specialization. Gone are the days of the single-handed doctor and the 'handmaiden' nurse. Instead we see a range of specialists with differing expertise dealing with patients at different stages of their lives, different stages of their conditions, and in different settings. Increasingly, patient services are being provided in the community as well as in hospitals. Within the traditional professions of medicine and nursing, training and additional qualifications have become necessary for advanced roles. New faculties, Royal Colleges and professional associations have arisen to validate and support members' interests. Newer professions (the therapists) have also developed, to attend to the rehabilitation of patients, while radiographers and geneticists/genetic counsellors are examples of those with expertise in the use and implications of diagnostic innovations.

Not surprisingly academics, politicians, professional organizations, senior managers and health professionals themselves have been much exercised by the perceived problems arising from such a complex organization, with much written about the implications for staff and patients and many solutions proposed. One major theme in the literature is that of the implications of recent policy changes for professional autonomy, an issue that has produced a continuing and lively debate particularly within the medical profession. Another area of concern for both professionals and managers responsible for organizing health services is the question of the changing pattern of skills required to provide an effective and efficient service and its relationship to the skills of the existing professionals.

Medical dominance and the other health care professions

THE PROFESSIONAL PROJECT

It has been argued (Freidson 1970) that one of the key characteristics of a profession, as opposed to other occupations, is that it is only the professions that have been deliberately granted autonomy, including the exclusive right to determine who can legitimately do their work and how that work should be done. Medicine has been seen as the paradigmatic profession, a 'publicly mandated and state-backed monopolistic supplier of a valued service, exercising autonomy in the workplace and collegiate control over recruitment, training and the regulation of members' conduct' (Elston 1991, p.58). Much of the early commentaries on professions focused on discussion of these traits. The doctor came to be seen as the 'ideal type' of a professional: someone with a vocation and commitment to help fellow human beings using a particular expertise based on a body of esoteric knowledge, who would always put the interests of the clients first and not seek to exploit their vulnerability. Attention then turned to the marketplace and the way medicine had succeeded in cornering the market for health care by driving unqualified healers out of business and achieving 'occupational closure', i.e. ensuring that doctors alone were responsible for selecting and training new recruits and regulating practice (see Armstrong 2000). The 1858 Medical Act, which established the General Council of Medical Education and Registration (known as the GMC), achieved this for doctors thereby ensuring the high status, autonomy and power that other health sector occupations subsequently aspired to and sought to emulate.

By the 1970s there was much greater scepticism about professionals' claims of beneficence and community orientation and much more interest in professional power and how it was exercised. Attention turned to 'professionalization' as a specific historical and political process and to the strategies and tactics (such as 'closure', which refers to actions employed by professions to control and limit their memberships) used with more or less success by occupational groups, such as nurses and the therapists, to gain control over the market for their services and/or to gain state support for occupational self-regulation (Freidson 1970; Larson 1977). Groups have also progressed their claims to professional status by attempting to define and formalize their independent knowledge bases, including by educating practitioners to degree level and engaging in research. To this end, seats of learning have been established; Tilley (2005), for instance, notes that Edinburgh University was the first institution in the UK to offer degrees to nurses. Manchester, King's College London and Cardiff were early followers, and by the end of the 1980s plans were afoot to educate all nurses to at least undergraduate diploma level (United Kingdom Central Council for Nursing, Midwifery and Health

Visiting 1986). At the time of writing the UK's regulatory body for nursing (the Nursing and Midwifery Council) is consulting on standards to support implementation of its historic decision that *all* future nurses should be degree-qualified at the point of registration. Physiotherapy, as a further example, became an all-graduate entry profession in 1992. Across both these, and other, aspirant groups great energy has also been put into developing profession-specific knowledge through research. Other actions taken by groups in support of their attempts to establish their credentials include the setting up of professional bodies, such as the Royal College of Nursing (established in 1916) and the Chartered Society for Physiotherapy (established in 1977).

'BOUNDARY WARS'

Instead of focusing on the projects or tactics of a single profession, or aspiring profession, attention was turned to the 'system of professions'. This stemmed from the proposition that the power of a profession lies in its jurisdiction and that each profession/occupation is linked to others, with the boundaries being constantly negotiated (Abbott 1988). While much of the rhetoric in policy documents and the professional literature emphasizes the importance of 'teamwork', in everyday practice the exact structure of the 'team', the distribution of responsibility and who has the power to lead/direct the team can often be unclear and the subject of dispute.

The ongoing debate has been carried out at both local and national level by the various stakeholders. There have also been a number of recent empirical studies, often using ethnographic methods, illustrating what has actually happened in a range of different settings in primary and secondary care and how the professionals involved perceive their situation and attempt to resolve problems (Carmel 2006; Grant *et al.* 2008; Sanders and Harrison 2007; Speed and Luker 2006). These illustrate different strategies by which doctors maintain their relative power, and ways in which the newer professions utilize a wider set of legitimacy claims as a means of strengthening their role and credibility within an increasingly fluid health care environment. Commentators have also pointed out that policymakers may aspire to a rather harmonious view of open knowledge-sharing within a community of practice, not recognizing that this may be difficult to achieve in the face of the significant power differentials in the NHS and the existing institutional realities. Knowledge-sharing is largely a voluntary exercise, characterized by informal social relations and, as such, is not amenable to control from executive management. Where a professional logic of specialization and hierarchy is dominant then relations between (and also within) professions remain essentially paternalistic and authoritarian: knowledge-sharing then tends to reflect or reinforce power differentials, with others deferring to (or resisting) the interests of doctors (see Currie and Suhomlinova 2006). If one of the characteristics of a professional is the possession of expert knowledge it is perhaps not surprising that, in order to protect their own position, individuals may be reluctant to share their expertise across professional boundaries.

DEPROFESSIONALIZATION

Such behaviour becomes even more likely in the context of rapid change and fluctuations in the supply of labour. By the 1990s concepts such as 'deprofessionalization' and 'proletarianization' began to appear in the literature. In the USA the gradual decline of medical dominance was attributed to the growing corporate and bureaucratic structure of American medicine. Increasingly, doctors were becoming salaried while power was passing from the profession to the large health corporations that composed the expanding medical industrial complex (McKinlay and Stoeckle 1988; Riska 2001). There has been considerable criticism and debate about the best way of theorizing such observable trends, their relevance to work situations as different as the USA and the UK, and the difficulties of defining and testing such concepts as 'deprofessionalization' and 'proletarianization'. Some have seen recent moves towards privatization and greater government involvement in quality improvement, standard-setting and professional regulation, as well as the imposition of new contracts, as marking a similar process for the UK. The undoubtedly heated debate continues, reflecting a variety of professional, political and managerial perspectives. What may be seen by health professionals, particularly doctors, as eroding professional power and autonomy may be seen by managers and politicians as necessary for service development and more effective and efficient health care (see Elston 1991; Ham and Alberti 2002). Policymakers may view the boundaries and distinctions between different professional groups as a positive hindrance to improving services, and recent examples of policy-driven changes to occupational roles are evident, including the extension of medication-prescribing to nurses and pharmacists.

The use of standards and frameworks, coupled with tighter regulation and the closer examination of performance, increase the likelihood of practice being constrained (Crinson 2005). Clinical guidelines, care pathways and other health technologies of this type carry the potential to shape everyday practice in powerful ways. Davies (2004), reflecting on the significance of these developments, observes that:

> Calls for a new kind of professionalism are now mounting and a number of organizational changes are under way. These changes include the incorporation into practice of clinical guidelines and protocols, designed both to support health professionals in keeping abreast of changing knowledge and to facilitate the breaking down of boundaries, the emergence of new hybrid practitioners and the implementation of direct appraisal of clinicians. Measures concerned with empowering patients to be at the heart of decisions about their own care and with abandoning the paternalism of an earlier era are also important. Above all, there is a stress not on 'clinical autonomy' but 'clinical accountability'. This means giving an account of the reasoning behind clinical decisions – in one-to-one settings with patients, in clinical governance arrangements and in wider arenas of audit and inspection. (p.59)

The workforce and the question of skill mix

So far we have mainly considered the health care system, the changes it has undergone and predictions about a possible future from the perspective of those professionals who are directly involved in delivering clinical services to patients. But NHS managers are professionals too. As noted above, their perspective is likely to be somewhat different since they are charged with implementing changing government policies and delivering services that represent good value for money with the resources allocated. Current social and demographic trends are likely to continue into the foreseeable future, with the ageing of the population and the rise in chronic diseases leading to greater demand for health care in both hospitals and the community. Shortages of professionals can arise in periods of expansion – as happened in the 1960s and again now – and can be met either by recruiting outside the UK or by initiatives involving delegation of tasks or extension of roles to other professionals or less-qualified care assistants.

OVERSEAS RECRUITMENT

Many countries are reporting shortages across a range of professions at a time of relatively high workforce mobility, and the use of the global market to fill such gaps is now a common recruitment strategy in many developed countries. The NHS is no exception, though international recruitment is now governed by a code of practice introduced in 2001, which requires NHS employers not to recruit from developing countries unless there is a government-to-government agreement that active recruitment is acceptable (in 2007 this only applied to China, India and the Philippines). In the years 2000–01 to 2003–04 the Philippines were the single most important non-UK source of nurses for the UK register.

In total, between April 1997 and March 2005 there was an aggregate total of more than 80,000 overseas nurses admitted to the UK register. In the early 1990s, overseas countries were the source of about one in ten nurses admitted to the register. In recent years, overseas countries have on average contributed approximately 45% of the annual number of new nurse entrants (Buchan 2006). Similar trends have been noted for doctors. Current estimates suggest that almost one-third of doctors practising in the NHS are from overseas and that the vast majority of these are from the Indian subcontinent. Policy initiatives recently developed bear a striking resemblance to what was being proposed in the 1960s, most notably the plan to expand the medical workforce through the active recruitment of overseas qualified doctors. The migration dynamics are changing, however, with many European Union trained doctors taking the place of those from the Indian subcontinent (Esmail 2007).

Traditionally overseas recruits have tended to fill gaps in the Cinderella specialities (for example, mental health and older people's services), and have found themselves working in the more deprived and/or industrial regions of the UK such as the South Wales valleys and inner cities. Skilled British health care professionals who have qualified in the UK also have the option of going abroad to North America, Australia or New Zealand as well as Europe and many do so in order to settle, particularly if job and further training opportunities in the UK are perceived as being restricted.

SKILL-MIX CHANGE

Moves towards even greater flexibility in the labour force will have obvious advantages for those responsible for managing the delivery of services in areas. Changing role boundaries within and between staff groups by extending, delegating and substituting existing roles, or by introducing new ones, is an attractive option and one that is being increasingly used in developed countries. In the UK, nurses are taking on tasks that were previously the preserve of doctors, such as medication-prescribing, and it has been suggested that an additional 74,000 health care assistants (HCAs) will be needed over the next 20 years (Bosley and Dale 2008; Wanless 2002). Most of the published research on HCAs is on their training or their role in hospital settings and a number of tensions and concerns around the nursing care skill-mix have been identified, which Bosley and Dale summarize as follows:

> Nurses claim professional identity on the basis of holistic, patient-centred care, as distinct from the task-oriented approach they attribute to HCAs. However, this distinction is contested by many HCAs who interact with and relate to patients in a way that nurses are increasingly unable to do. Nurses report experiencing 'role deprivation' at the loss of relationships with patients and hands-on care. Some defend their identity by treating HCAs as subordinates, highlighting professional credentials, and referring to professional accountability and their knowledge as a basis for a different approach to activities that are also performed by HCAs. Nurses may undervalue HCAs' experience, skills, and knowledge of local community and organization, and restrict their involvement in higher level activities. Despite their less powerful position, there is evidence that HCAs also engage in boundary-work, by exerting influence over less-experienced staff and choosing whether to share or withhold patient and organizational knowledge depending on their relationship with individual nurses. Such activities are not conducive to effective team work or patient care. (Bosley and Dale 2008, p.120)

Such findings have implications for teamwork, quality of care and patient safety. Moreover, as Doyal and Cameron (2000) point out, new integrated mechanisms of workforce planning will be required, and significant problems are likely to arise if the 'core' skills and responsibilities of the different groups change and the organization of the NHS labour force becomes increasingly out of line with the traditional map of the health professions. They argue that the resulting tensions will not be amenable to solutions devised by individual directorates or trusts, or by the different professional bodies working alone. Indeed, in the case of the allied health professions, unilateral decisions taken by professional bodies to tighten entry qualifications could be seen as artificially restricting supply and hence improving career prospects, as happened in the 1980s (see Dyson 1990).

Given the importance of the topic, there is a striking lack of research on changing the skill-mix of the NHS workforce, particularly role changes involving workers other than doctors and nurses. Having undertaken a systematic review of the evidence in this area, Sibbald, Shen and McBride (2004) comment that:

> Cost-effectiveness was generally not evaluated, nor was the wider impact of the change on health care systems... In order to make informed choices, health care planners need good research evidence about the likely consequences of skill-mix change. The findings from existing research need to be made more accessible while the dearth of evidence makes new research necessary. (p.28)

McPherson et al. (2006) looked at evidence about extended roles for allied health professionals and concluded that there was little evidence as to how best to introduce such roles, or how best to educate, support and mentor practitioners. Given the pressures arising from professional mobility (whether planned or not) and the need to meet gaps in the service, it is not surprising that managers will seek greater flexibility among those at their disposal but it appears that such changes have the potential to create considerable difficulties for the professionals involved – possibly leading to a clash of values and the detriment of patient care.

INTERPROFESSIONAL EDUCATION: THE ANSWER TO THE PROBLEM?

As Finch (2000, pp.1138–1139) comments, the NHS wants students to be prepared for interprofessional working in any or all of the following senses:

- To 'know about' the roles of other professional groups.

- To be able to 'work with' other professionals, in the context of a team where each member has a clearly defined role.

- To be able to 'substitute for' roles traditionally played by other professionals, when circumstances suggest that this would be more effective.

- To provide flexibility in career routes: 'moving across'.

Speaking from her position as the vice-chancellor of a higher education institution, Finch points out that, while universities and colleges are eager to work with the health service, they do require greater clarity about objectives. Moreover, different types of education provision are required, depending on which of the four versions of 'interprofessional' is being advocated. Her view was that it would be much more productive to invite higher education institutions to produce proposals to support the kind of career flexibility that the NHS desires, than to prescribe the form that this should take, e.g. a common foundation programme.

This seems reasonable, given the, again, very limited research base available on the effects of interprofessional education initiatives on professional practice and health care outcomes (see Reeves *et al.* 2008). Very few studies were found for inclusion in this systematic review, and many were described by Reeves *et al.* as 'not of high quality', leading the authors to the conclusion that there can be no certainty regarding the effect of interprofessional education or the key features of interprofessional training that enable professionals to work effectively together.

CONCLUSIONS

This short overview of the way in which health care organization and delivery has changed over time, and intertwined with wider social and other changes, has, we hope, convinced the reader that, however one might characterize the current state of affairs, it is unlikely to remain the same for very long. Who can say with certainty, for example, what the implications of global economic crisis will be for future patterns of health care organization and delivery?

One of the most striking features of the past two hundred years has been the steady rise of doctors to a position of increasing power and prestige, such that the physician became the epitome of the professional person and the benchmark for theorizing about professions and professionalization in general. In the case of the doctor this role has also been associated with notions of a special vocation and altruism in that he (and, historically, it usually was a man) is expected and trusted to put the patient's interests first. Thus, a service ideal and an esoteric knowledge base came to be seen as the basis of any profession in society. However, as the sociology of medicine developed in the 1960s sociologists began re-examining the role of the medical profession in society and its claims, and, in particular, to enquire exactly how this profession had managed to become so powerful by the mid-twentieth century while at the same time managing to persuade the general public that such power was in the public interest. In other words, how exactly had the profession managed to pull this off (see Armstrong 2000)?

We have also shown the degree to which this state of affairs has changed. Increasing specialization between and within occupations, technological advances, deskilling, the rise of new health care groups, managers with remits to make binding decisions and a lay public now willing to challenge traditional authority are some of the forces coalescing to alter this landscape radically (Elston 1991). Small wonder, then, that the professions can be found talking up their contributions, lest − like the remedial gymnasts who became submerged within the profession of physiotherapy − they disappear altogether. And what of the purpose and place of values in this context? It may be, as Stephen Pattison and Huw Thomas hint in this book's Introduction, that it is precisely in circumstances of this type that professions invoke 'values' as a means of bolstering their claims.

And what of the practitioner: the individual professional who, whilst caught up in the maelstrom, is still called on to give of his or her best in the day-in, day-out, health care encounter? In his most recent work on professionalism, Freidson (2001) argues that the position of professionals in society today is being seriously weakened in the name of competition and efficiency and that, on the contrary, monopoly and also freedom of judgement or discretion in performance are essential to those occupations we term 'professions'. His aim is to present a 'model of the logic of professionalism that can enjoy the same privileged intellectual status as the logics of the market and the firm' (p.4). In his view, clarification of the principles underlying professions will provide them with a more adequate defence against those of the market (that celebrates competition and cost) and those of the firm (that invokes the virtue of efficiency through standardization). (As we have seen, both these latter models have played an increasingly important part in UK policy and health sector organizations.)

Looking into the future, Freidson (2001) suggests that the worst, and not unlikely, possibility is that professionals will slowly be transformed into especially privileged technical workers operating within boundaries, channels and goals carefully established by their employers. He anticipates a trend toward a two-tier professional system composed of a permanent, relatively small, élite corps of professionals who do research and set standards of performance in practice organizations and an often floating population of qualified practitioners who may be employed on a temporary and sometimes part-time basis. Efforts to standardize the work of the rank-and-file professionals will increase in order to reduce cost and achieve better control and supervision. Such standardization will involve authoritative professional knowledge provided partly by the professional cadre in the organization and also by national élites empowered to create binding rules to govern the work of practitioners. Disciplinary control of professional training is likely to narrow, with curricula responding more to the tasks required by employers. Within each profession the gap in income between the rank-and-file and the élite in supervisory and consulting specialist positions will almost certainly become greater, as will tension and possible conflict between them, but all will remain recognizable 'professionals'.

Among the likely consequences of this might be a decline in the quality of service to individual clients due to the minimization of discretion in everyday practice, resulting, in turn, in reduced job satisfaction of the ordinary practitioner. The emphasis on the practical needs of the State and the satisfaction of what the public believes to be its needs may restrict the development of knowledge and risks the professions losing their 'freedom to set their own agenda for the development of their discipline and assume responsibility for its use' (p.213). In reading the following chapters the reader is invited to judge the relevance of Freidson's predictions and their implications.

REFERENCES

6, P. and Peck, E. (2004) 'Modernization: the ten commitments of New Labour's approach to public management?' *International Public Management Journal 7*, 1, 1–18.

Abbott, A. (1988) *The System of Professions: An Essay on the Division of Expert Labor.* Chicago, IL: University of Chicago Press.

Albrecht, G.L., Fitzpatrick, R. and Scrimshaw, S. (eds) (2000) *The Handbook of Social Studies in Health and Medicine.* London: Sage.

Allsop, J. (1984) *Health Policy and the National Health Service.* London: Longman.

Armstrong, D. (2000) 'Social Theorising about Health and Illness.' In G.L. Albrecht, R. Fitzpatrick and S. Scrimshaw (eds) *The Handbook of Social Studies in Health and Medicine.* London: Sage.

Bosley, S. and Dale, J. (2008) 'Health care assistants in General practice: practical and conceptual issues of skill-mix change.' *British Journal of General practice 58*, 547, 118–124.

Buchan, J. (2006) 'Filipino nurses in the UK: a case study in active international recruitment.' *Harvard Health Policy Review 7*, 1, 113–120.

Carmel, S. (2006) 'Boundaries obscured and boundaries reinforced: incorporation as a strategy of occupational enhancement for intensive care.' *Sociology of Health and Illness 28*, 2, 154–177.

Crinson, I. (2005) 'The direction of health policy in New Labour's third term.' *Critical Social Policy 25*, 4, 507–516.

Currie, G. and Suhomlinova, O. (2006) 'The impact of institutional forces upon knowledge-sharing in the UK NHS: the triumph of professional power and the inconsistency of policy.' *Public Administration 84*, 1, 1–30.

Davies, C. (2004) 'Regulating the health care workforce: next steps for research.' *Journal of Health Services Research and Policy 9*, Supplement 1, 55–61.

Department of Health (1989) *Working for Patients.* London: HMSO.

Department of Health (2000) *The NHS Plan: A Plan for Investment, a Plan for Reform.* London: Department of Health.

Department of Health (2005) *Staff in the NHS 2004: An Overview of Staff Numbers.* London: Department of Health.

Dingwall, R., Rafferty, A.M., Webster, C. (1998) *An Introduction to the Social History of Nursing.* London: Routledge.

Dixon, J. (2001) 'Transforming the NHS: what chance for the new government?' *Economic Affairs 21*, 4, 4–8.

Doyal, L. and Cameron, A. (2000) 'Reshaping the NHS workforce.' *British Medical Journal 320*, 7241, 1023–1024.

Dyson, R. (1990) 'Shortage of therapists.' *British Medical Journal 300*, 6716, 4.

Elston, M. (1991) 'The Politics of Professional Power: Medicine in a Changing Health Service.' In J. Gabe, M. Calnan and M. Bury (eds) *The Sociology of the Health Service.* London: Routledge.

Esmail, A. (2007) 'Asian doctors in the NHS: service and betrayal.' *British Journal of General practice 57*, 543, 827–834.

Evans, D. (2004) 'Shifting the balance of power? UK public health policy and capacity building.' *Critical Public Health 14*, 1, 63–75.

Finch, J. (2000) 'Interprofessional education and teamworking: a view from the education providers.' *British Medical Journal 321*, 7269, 1138–1140.

Freidson, E. (1970) *Profession of Medicine: A Study of the Sociology of Applied Knowledge.* New York: Harper and Row.

Freidson, E. (2001) *Professionalism: The Third Logic.* Cambridge: Polity Press.

Grant, S., Huby, G., Watkins, F., Checkland, K., McDonald, R., Davies, H. and Guthrie, B. (2008) 'The impact of pay-for-performance on professional boundaries in UK General practice: an ethnographic study.' *Sociology of Health and Illness 31*, 2, 229–245.

Greener, I. (2004) 'The three moments of New Labour's health policy discourse.' *Policy and Politics 32*, 3, 303–316.

Griffiths, R. (1983) *NHS Management Inquiry*. London: Department of Health and Social Security.

Ham, C. (1996) 'Managed markets in health care: the UK Experiment.' *Health Policy 35*, 3, 279–292.

Ham, C. and Alberti, K.G.M.M. (2002) 'The medical profession, the public, and the government.' *British Medical Journal 324*, 7341, 838–842.

Hood, C. (1991) 'A public management for all seasons?' *Public Administration 69*, Spring, 3–19.

Klein, R. (1983) *The Politics of the National Health Service*. London: Longman.

Klein, R. (1998) 'Why Britain is reorganizing its National Health Service – yet again.' *Health Affairs 17*, 4, 111–125.

Larson, M.S. (1977) *The Rise of Professionalism*. Berkeley, CA: University of California Press.

Le Grand, J. (1999) 'Competition, cooperation, or control? Tales from the British National Health Service.' *Health Affairs 18*, 3, 27–39.

Levitt, R. (1979) *The Reorganised National Health Service*. London: Croom Helm.

McKinlay, J. and Stoeckle, J. (1988) 'Corporatization and the social transformation of doctoring.' *International Journal of Health Services 18*, 2, 191–205.

McPherson, K., Kersten, P., George, S., Lattimer, V., Breton, A., Ellis, B., Kaur, D. and Frampton, G. (2006) 'A systematic review of evidence about extended roles for allied health professionals.' *Journal of Health Services Research and Policy 11*, 4, 240–247.

Pill, R., Wainwright, P., McNamee, M. and Pattison, S. (2004) 'Understanding Professions and Professionals in the Context of Values.' In S. Pattison and R. Pill (eds) *Values in Professional Practice: Lessons for Health, Social care and Other Professionals*. Oxford: Radcliffe.

Porter, R. (1996) *Cambridge Illustrated History of Medicine*. Cambridge: Cambridge University Press.

Porter, R. (1997) *The Greatest Benefit to Mankind: a Medical History of Mankind from Antiquity to the Present*. London: Harper Collins.

Powell, M. (2000) 'Analysing the "New" British National Health Service.' *International Journal of Health Planning and Management 15*, 2, 89–101.

Reeves, S., Zwarenstein, M., Goldman, J., Barr, H., Freeth, D., Hammick, M. and Koppel, I. (2008) '*Interprofessional Education: Effects on Professional Practice and Health Care Outcomes.*' Cochrane Database of Systematic Reviews, Issue 1. Art. No.: CD002213. DOI: 10.1002/14651858.CD002213.pub2.

Riska, E. (2001) 'Health Professions and Occupations.' In W. Cockerham (ed.) *The Blackwell Companion to Medical Sociology*. Oxford: Blackwell.

Sanders, T. and Harrison, S. (2007) 'Professional legitimacy claims in the multidisciplinary workplace: the case of heart failure care.' *Sociology of Health and Illness 30*, 2, 289–308.

Sibbald, B., Shen, J. and McBride, A. (2004) 'Changing the skill-mix of the health care work force.' *Journal of Health Services Research and Policy 9*, 1, 28–38.

Speed, S. and Luker, K. (2006) 'Getting a visit: how district nurses and general practitioners "organise" each other in primary care.' *Sociology of Health and Illness 28*, 7, 883–902.

Stacey, M. (1988) *The Sociology of Health and Healing*. London: Unwin Hyman.

Tilley, S. (2005) 'Fragile Tradition: Institutionalisation of Knowledge of Psychiatric and Mental Health Nursing in the Department of Nursing Studies, the University of Edinburgh.' In S. Tilley (ed.) *Psychiatric and Mental Health Nursing: The Field of Knowledge*. Oxford: Blackwell.

United Kingdom Central Council for Nursing, Midwifery and Health Visiting (1986) *Project 2000: A New Preparation for Practice*. London: UKCC.

Wanless, D. (2002) *Securing our Future Health: Taking a Long-Term View. Final Report*. London: HM Treasury.

Chapter 2

Why Do Changes in Society and Institutions Matter for Professional Values?

Andrew Edgar

INTRODUCTION

The purpose of this chapter is to provide a sketch of the policy and theoretical context within which health care professions have worked in the post-war period. It will be suggested that professions' self-understanding, and the values that they embrace, have to have been shaped by this context. The perspective adopted is very much that of a social philosopher – that is to say that underpinning the following narrative is a concern with the manner in which the understanding of the key roles within health care is articulated, and more broadly, how issues of social justice are incorporated into debates and policy decisions over health care.

The following narrative will seek to explore three themes. First, it will sketch the changes in the relationships between the professional, the patient or client and the State. Centrally, it will be suggested that the balance between the responsibility of the individual for their own health and wellbeing and the scope of the State's support for that individual, has been regularly rethought. Second, the patient's experience of illness and disease, and their treatment, have undergone changes and critical reappraisals throughout the period. It will be suggested that this entails new evaluations of the nature and worth of health care practice, that in turn impact upon the professional's self-understanding. Finally, and most importantly, the narrative presented here is one of a growing suspicion of the legitimacy of the power that the professional wields. The assumption that professionals have a more or less unquestioned autonomy and control over their patients is challenged variously and with a corrosive subtlety. Part of this narrative focuses on the fact that the professions find themselves confronted by an increasingly well-informed, articulate and assertive clientele. This phenomenon is complemented by the increasing regulation of professions, and their constraint within administrative and monitoring systems over which they have little or no control. Such systems serve, to a significant degree, to define the profession or curtail the scope of its self-understanding, as well as potentially undermining its self-confidence and self-esteem. The understanding and legitimation of the power of professions therefore lies at the core of this account.

It will be assumed that the post-war history of the National Health Service (NHS) and the welfare state can be divided into three broadly understood periods. Each period is characterized by a different fundamental philosophy underpinning its approach to social policy, albeit that actual practice may be much more complex and ambiguous. The first period would begin with the initiation of the modern welfare state in the 1940s. In response to Beveridge's five giants – want, disease, ignorance, squalor and idleness – the welfare state offered 'cradle to grave' protection to the citizen. This was linked to the then dominance of Keynesian economics, and thus to the State management of the economy to ensure steady economic growth and high levels of employment. The values associated with such policy can, at least in its initial period, be understood in terms of communal solidarity: the society as a whole bears a burden of responsibility to the wellbeing of all its members.

This approach to social policy breaks down decisively in the 1970s. The apparent failure of Keynesian economics (in the stagflation of the mid- to late 1970s) opens the way to more neo-classical approaches to economic management, and the rise of libertarian ideologies and the New Right (see Chapter 1 above for an account of New Right ideas in action during the years of Conservative administration from 1979 onwards). Values shift from communal concern to an emphasis on individual autonomy. The 1990s see the rise of a 'Third Way' (Giddens 1998) that strives to correct both the paternalistic extremes of the original welfare state, and the dangers of inequality and marginalization that occur within a free market. This approach takes a more communal view of the citizen and patient – as having responsibilities as well as rights, and whose participation in policymaking and health care provision is articulated through involvement in on-going debates and the formulation of personal and public opinion. These three periods, and the fate of professional self-understanding within each of them, will now be examined in more detail.

THE WELFARE STATE

The early development of the NHS and a comprehensive welfare state strictly falls outside of the scope of most of the essays in this book. However, precisely in so far as this period yields an image of welfare provision for which there is either nostalgic yearning or a critical reaction, it is crucial to shaping any understanding of later developments.

The vision of a welfare state provided by Beveridge, alongside Bevan's of a national health service, offered the promise of the removal of social inequalities, including those created through unequal access to health care. The State took responsibility for the individual, protecting him or her against the misfortunes of unemployment, old age, and illness, and thereby in Beveridge's words, making 'want under any circumstances unnecessary' (Beveridge 1942, para.17). Funding for this welfare state came from a flat-rate national insurance payment, contributed by all employers and employees. Yet, as Fink's overview of the period argues, there are already compromises and tensions within this vision. The responsibility of the State to support the individual citizen cannot be pursued at the cost of the individual's responsibility for his or her own life and family, or his or her duty to contribute to the community as a whole. This led to low welfare payments, beneath subsistence levels, and the more or less explicit articulation of some distinction between the deserving and undeserving poor (Fink 2005). In the context of welfare provision, this distinction is articulated in terms of the presupposition of full employment, so that the non-worker (who does not make national insurance contributions) loses the right to full benefits. Further, it is assumed that this worker is typically male, providing for a wife and family. Women are thus denied welfare payments other than those provided through their male supporter.

While such assumptions are less relevant to the provision of health care, there are nonetheless certain implicit assumptions about the nature of the patient, of disease and illness, and of the professional carer incorporated within the NHS. The doctor, beginning at the level of the general practitioner (GP), plays a crucial role as the gatekeeper to the service, and thus in the determination of who deserves treatment. A largely unquestioned trust in the doctor, and the assumption of their professional integrity and autonomy, grounded the early NHS. Within the sociology of this period, this image of the professional is reinforced – not least through study of the health care professions, albeit that much of this research originates in America, not the UK. At the centre of this analysis lies sociologist Talcott Parsons' work. For Parsons, the authority of the professional comes through their access to an expert knowledge base. While Parsons was not blind to the commercial implications of professional occupations, he argues that the professional's morality places him or her as an altruistic servant of their clients, in contrast to the more self-interested approach of the 'business man' (Parsons 1949). In addition, the prestige of the professional is seen to arise from their association with the core values of the society.

This image of the medical professional is complemented by images of disease and the patient. Parsons' theory of the sick role takes as its norm the experience of acute illness. A person falls ill and so is unable to pursue their usual social activities (or roles). The illness legitimates the person's withdrawal from routine activity and permits a retreat into a sick role, where the normal obligations to one's work and other roles are suspended. The sick role is not without its own obligations, however. The sick person is obliged to do what they can to recover, and this entails, not least, complying with the expert advice of medical professionals. Upon recovery, the person returns to mundane life, in relation to which the period of illness is treated as a mere hiatus (Parsons 1951). If the sick role does indeed articulate the implicit assumptions that govern medical practice during this period, then it is not simply its focus upon the acute nature of illness that is significant.

Crucially, the patient is understood very much as an individual, and the experience of illness is not interpreted in relationship to the patient's social context (whether that be the family, work or the wider environment). At this early stage, public health remained the remit of local authorities, not the regional hospital boards or the executive councils that supervised general practices. In addition, it can be suggested that the sick role presents health care provision as having a highly instrumental role within the economy. The grounding motivation for providing universal access to health care is that it facilitates the speedy and efficient return of workers to the workplace (and, by extension, if workers are predominantly male, the return of women to their necessary supportive roles within the home). This is unsurprising, given the fact that the funding of the NHS and welfare state as a whole relied upon the contributions of those in work (and, indeed, upon high rates of employment in general).

The breakdown of these conceptions of professionalism and of health care are charted in the development of sociology. A group of sociologists who became known as the social interactionists began, in the 1950s and 1960s, to question what Parsons takes to be more or less self-evident about the grounding of professional status in the professional's expertise and its commitment to core social values. Sociologists such as Hughes question the distinctive nature of the professional knowledge base, arguing that the profession is not readily distinguished from any other occupational group. Hughes suggests rather that the status of the profession is achieved through quite separate processes of social negotiation (Hughes 1958). Similarly, Freidson (1970) was to argue that the power of the medical profession lay in its actively militating, through representative groups such as the British Medical Association (BMA) in the UK, to preserve its status and position. The representative bodies of the profession are thereby seen to work, not altruistically as Parsons supposes, but in order to safeguard the interests of the profession's members (see Millerson 1964). Such accounts are complemented and magnified by criticisms of the 'medicalization' of society. Thinkers such as Illich (1976), and, also within a different tradition, Foucault (1973) as well as sociologists such as Oakley (1981), began to see medicine not as solving problems but as the source of problems, precisely in so far as an excessive range of problems were treated as being medical, with the subsequent treatment leading to adverse side-effects and to the chronic dependence of the patient upon medical care.

Such accounts may be taken as marking a growing scepticism about professional power (not merely within academia, but also within the wider population) and thus the trust that should be invested in the profession. The authority of the medical professional is increasingly undermined by a change in the nature of the patient in the post-war period. The expansion of the middle classes, attended as it was by an expansion of universal education, entailed that the doctor was increasingly confronted by a well-educated and articulate patient, and a patient who was potentially the doctor's social equal. It may be suggested that such patients – and such patients who are also citizens and taxpayers – take less kindly to the paternalism and collectivism that lay at the heart of the original conception of the welfare state.

A further, but important, dimension of an increasing challenge to the power of the professional is expressed in the rise of medical ethics. In this case, the challenge to the professional can be seen to arise simultaneously with the establishment of the NHS, in so far as the major stimulus to modern medical ethics came from the revelation of Nazi medical atrocities and the subsequent Nuremberg Code (1947), the Declaration of Geneva (1948) and the Helsinki Declaration (1964). The post-war period sees individual professions develop their own codes of conduct or codes of ethics. The precise purpose of such codes can be debated, not least as to whether they are codes of conduct (and thus the quasi-legal documents through which the profession polices its members) or codes of ethics proper that offer guidance and encourage personal development in the face of moral dilemmas. Yet the mere existence of such codes suggests a growing willingness within professions to reflect upon and articulate the professional altruism that Parsons took largely on trust.

Beyond the articulation of ethical codes, the development of principlism (in particular in America) can be taken as the key formulation of medical ethics in its first stage of maturation. This is the case not least because principlism places the interests of the patient at the centre of medical concerns. The principlist approach seeks to bring together two major approaches to ethics: consequentialism (that looks to the good and bad consequences of any action in order to assess its moral worth); and deontology (that looks to the rights, duties and obligations of people). This leads to a formulation of four principles that should guide moral decision-making (see Beauchamp and Childress 1979). These principles are those of beneficence, non-maleficence, autonomy and justice. The first two promote consequentialist notions, in that the physician should do good and avoid unnecessary harm (which is itself a recognition of the dangers of medicine). It is the principles of autonomy and justice that pose the major challenge to the paternalistic authority of the physician. Respect for the autonomy of the patient entails, crucially, a recognition of the importance of the patient giving informed consent to any treatment (and in the light of the Nazi experience, consent to involvement in medical research), and the protection of confidentiality. Furthermore, it can be suggested that in recognizing the importance of autonomy, the medical profession acknowledges that it now works with a patient body that has typically higher educational attainment. The principle of autonomy is expressive of a patient who need no longer tolerate medical paternalism passively. Justice, the fourth principle, demands that different patients are treated equitably, and thus that discrimination between patients on non-medical grounds is unacceptable. Medical ethics in general, and principlism in particular, thereby, begin to establish the position of the patient as a partner in their treatment, rather than as a merely passive recipient.

THE NEW RIGHT

The original conception of the welfare state was confronted by regular challenges prior to the 1970s. The welfare state as a whole had failed to remove social inequality, as Abel-Smith and Townsend (1965) demonstrated, in contradiction to Rowntree's earlier and far more positive report on improving conditions in York (Rowntree and Lavers 1951). Subsequently the so-called Black Report would similarly serve to expose inequalities in health (Black *et al.* 1980; Townsend 1979). In addition, it can be suggested that the welfare state never enjoyed the wholehearted support of all the population. Crucially, amongst those it was most explicitly intended to serve, there remained both an ignorance to the rights that one held as a claimant upon the State, and a reluctance to exercise them. A stigma continued to be associated with the means testing that determined access to many forms of benefit, but also through an association between state welfare provision and charity (Fink 2005). The social consensus that was required to found the welfare state was thus under serious threat by the 1970s. Crucially, the 1970s also saw the erosion of its material base. The original conception of the welfare state presupposed full employment. Rising unemployment after the global economic crises of the early 1970s threatened that basis. The welfare state, and with it health care provision, were thus open to a radical rethinking.

The dominant form that this rethinking took was inspired by libertarian or New Right approaches to political philosophy and economics. At the core of this lay a commitment to respecting the autonomy of the individual, and thus to enabling individual choice, even in matters of welfare. The market offered a model for institutions that enable such choice, because buyers and sellers will come to a market free to make the economic decisions that they see as being most in line with their best interests. State restrictions on markets, precisely in so far as they remove freedom of choice from the buyer or seller, are thus seen as inhibiting autonomy. From this perspective even income tax can be seen to be morally illegitimate, precisely because it prevents the earner of that taxed income spending the money on their own behalf. The decision as to what the money should be spent upon is appropriated by the government (see Nozick 1974).

Within New Right thinking the market is seen as being the most efficient way of distributing resources because it bypasses the bureaucracy that is entailed in any form of state planning. A state is not required to anticipate and plan for the needs of its population. This shift in political philosophy provides a first and crucial step in legitimating the privatization of medical provision. A free market, divorced from state direction, allows individuals to choose to satisfy whatever needs can be covered by the income and capital available to them. Such thinking appealed to the perception that the welfare state was bureaucratic and inefficient, and, crucially, did so in a time when the scarcity of resources to fund welfare and particularly health provision was seemingly growing more pressing. Even if, in practice, the New Right did not bring about the abolition of the welfare state or the NHS, it did promise a more streamlined and thus less expensive system, with the introduction of market mechanisms (including an internal market within the NHS) and greater contributions from the private sector to the provision of welfare.

In practice, the transition between the old universalistic welfare state and the later conception was not the radical break that the shift in moral and political thought might suggest (see Mohan 2002). However, within health care it can be seen as inspiring a new conception of the patient: as consumer and rights holder. While the old welfare state, for the largely pragmatic reasons suggested above, situated its clients within male-dominated family units, in practice the patient was conceived as an individual. The New Right reinforced this individualistic conception, conceptualizing the patient as divorced from the care and support of their families, and thus failing to appreciate the impact that illness might have upon those associated with the immediate patient. The introduction of the Patient's Charter in 1991, which effectively summarized and publicized the patient's existing rights with respect to the NHS, served as a key articulation of this conception. This shift in the understanding of the patient, and the potential transformation of them into a consumer, also throws into question the understanding of health care. Potentially, health care becomes one more consumer commodity that can be distributed through the market (Spicker 1995). The special status of health care, as something worthy of moral rather than merely commercial concern, is questioned. Health itself, in this conception, becomes a mere commodity that one possesses and, like other commodities, it is something that one may insure. If damaged or lost, insurance will pay for its repair and replacement (Seedhouse 1986). Such conceptions, while obviously highly contested, nonetheless serve to redefine the patient's relationship to, and indeed responsibility for, their health, as well as further undermining the legitimacy of state provision of health care. If health care is merely one more commodity, then not only may it be produced and distributed through the private sector, but also decisions as to the appropriate health care for an individual will, ultimately, rest upon the consumer preferences of that individual.

While the original conception of the welfare state presupposes that health inequalities have a significant relationship with social inequalities, and that this is a matter of moral and political concern, the New Right conception, at its extreme, sees no difference between a person's inability to pay for health care and their inability to pay for a larger house or more expensive car. Potentially, those deserving health care are either those who can pay for it, or are those who have had the morally commendable foresight to insure and save against the future threat of illness. Significantly, such conceptions also challenge the position and status of the health care professional. Their expertise becomes a marketable commodity, and the value of that commodity lies, not in their own estimation of it, but in that of the patient-consumer. New Right thinking thereby further serves to wrest power away from the medical professions. In more practical terms, this is expressed in the NHS's internal market, where health authorities become purchasers of services from health care providers. The health authorities act on behalf of the consumer-patient, so that the provision of health care comes to be dictated by the perceived health care needs of the health authority's population, and not by the preferences and desires of the health care professional.

This changing understanding of the patient is complemented in a complex manner by the rise of health economics, and in particular the 'quality of life' movement. The cost of providing health care, and thus the funding of the NHS in real terms, had risen annually since 1948. This is typically attributed to rising demand that is stimulated by falling death rates, to increased expectations of what health care can and should deliver in terms of treatment, and to the exponential increase in the cost of new medical technologies and rising labour costs within the NHS. There is thus a perpetual perception of a resourcing crisis within the NHS (Lowe 2004). Health economics becomes important in the late 1970s and 1980s as a way of establishing the cost-efficiency of health services, and thus as a means for prioritizing (or, indeed, rationing) services. Crucially, by focusing on quality of life, health economists avoided the danger of treating health instrumentally, and merely as a resource that contributed to the broader economic efficiency of the society. Health is not given a monetary value, although the resources required to treat illness, disease and disability are. What matters about health is its value to the healthy person. The quality of life movement can thereby be seen as reinforcing the anti-paternalism that grounds other changes in this period. In order to determine the value of treatments in terms of their impact upon quality of life, relevant populations of patients or potential patients are surveyed. It is their evaluations of the worth of health, and indeed their very understanding of what health means to them, that are incorporated into the economic calculations, not those of the medical profession (see Bowling 1997; Hunt, McEwen and McKenna 1986).

In the early 1990s, the state of Oregon responded in a novel way to both the problem of scarce health care resources and that of public involvement in determining health care provision (Kirk 1993). Confronted by the failings of the federal Medicaid programme in the United States (which is to say, state provision of health care to the poorest individuals and families), the state of Oregon planned a fundamental revision of this programme. At the core of this plan lay the use of quality of life measures to rank the cost-effectiveness of different treatments. Once treatments had been prioritized, a decision could be made, given knowledge of available funds, as to which treatments would be funded, and which not. Scarce resources would be focused upon the most cost-effective treatments, in an overt act of rationing. Importantly, a second plank of the Oregon plan lay in a process of public consultation, through which 'community values' were elicited, and these values served to shape and modify the prioritization process. Thus, although rationing would take place, and certain treatments would not be available, that denial of treatment was legitimated in the moral choices of the community.

Although the Oregon experiment faced much criticism and opposition, it can be seen as having had an enormous influence upon thinking about health care globally. Crucially, in the UK, it set in train a multiplicity of public consultation processes, through which health authorities were expected to elicit and respond to the views of the public on health care and prioritization (see Bowling 1993). While this may, again, be seen as reinforcing the anti-paternalism of the period, ironically, in the context of the dominance of the New Right, it represented a shift away from the highly individualistic presuppositions of the libertarian. In effect, it heralded a further rethinking of what it means to be a patient, and thus of the relationship between patient and doctor. The patient ceases to be a mere consumer, and becomes, instead, a citizen, who has a responsibility to be involved in determining the nature and priorities of health care. This responsibility is exercised by engaging in informed dialogue with politicians and the professional providers. It is this vision that increasingly informs the final stage in the development of post-war social policy, that of the Third Way.

THE THIRD WAY

While the New Right can be regarded as having responded to real short-comings in the original conception of the welfare state, its perceived insensitivity towards the ability of the poor and deprived to provide for their own care resulted in an exacerbation of social inequality (Graham 2001). The initial vision that the New Labour government had for the NHS stresses that health care should be allocated according to 'need and need alone' (Department of Health 1997, para.2.13). While there remained something problematic in this resolution of problems of allocation purely in terms of a recognition of clinical need, the statement does protest against the intrusion of morally irrelevant factors into health care provision, such as ability to pay and geographical location (see Department of Health 2009, p.3). The social democracy of the Third Way can be characterized in terms of its continuing rejection of the 'one size fits all' mentality of the original welfare state. While a tolerance for privately funded provision of health care and welfare remains, in contrast to the New Right, there is a much greater scepticism as to the power and efficacy of the market, not least in its ability to serve a diversity of needs or to shape services to individual clients. This scepticism is grounded in a greater awareness of the dimensions of social inequality that structure the lives of individuals, and the implications that social relationships might have for an individual's health status, as well as the way in which social and cultural contexts might serve to constrain personal choice and bring about exclusion from social advantages. The individual citizen, and thus the recipient of welfare and health care, is situated in terms of hierarchies of class, gender, ethnicity, sexuality and age, for example, as well as within a richer family, social and cultural context. The task of governing becomes that of enabling the freedom of individuals, precisely by challenging and removing both the material and cultural impediments to full social participation that such hierarchies perpetuate. The personal autonomy that the New Right took for granted is thus now understood as something fragile and vulnerable that has to be actively realized and supported by the State.

The Third Way can therefore be seen as having taken up the conception of the patient suggested by the Oregon experiment, but in a more radical way. Oregon presupposed that citizens had values and views on health care that they could articulate. In practice, participants in the community meetings designed to elicit those values were overwhelmingly medical professionals, and not the people Medicare is designed to serve. Other countries, and most noticeably New Zealand, offered exercises that developed citizens' thinking about the problems and nature of rationing, before eliciting values or asking for priorities (Campbell 1995). One can argue that Third Way thinking has extended this, so that the citizen-patient is not merely expected to be involved in discussions about health care planning on the large scale, but also (and crucially for their relationship with medical professionals) in their use of health care services. The patient thereby becomes a responsible participant in their own treatment, and, indeed, in protecting and fostering their own health and wellbeing. This is manifest in programmes such as the promotion of healthy lifestyles, government provision of guidance on nutrition, and support to cease smoking. Significantly, the Expert Patient programme also recognized the shifting nature of illness itself (Department of Health 2001). The Parsonian sick role, noted above, presupposes that illness is normally acute. In practice, thanks in part to developments in medicine itself, it is chronic illness that is becoming increasingly prevalent (see Frank 1997). One does not now typically fall ill, take one's medicine and so recover. Chronic conditions, such as arthritis, may increase in prevalence thanks to longer life expectancy. New medical processes, including transplant programmes, require sustained medical interventions after the initial treatment, thereby permanently medicalizing the patient. Other conditions, such as cancers, may not be cured, but merely go into remission. The notion of the 'Expert Patient' recognizes this, at least in so far as it recognizes the advantages of the chronically-ill patient being better informed about their condition and so able to take responsibility for managing it.

The image of the involved and responsible patient can be seen as being articulated in the NHS Constitution. This document summarizes the legal rights of the patient, including the patient's 'right to make choices about [their] NHS care' (Department of Health 2009, p.7). But, the NHS will also 'strive to work in partnership' with patients (p.7), and those patients are ascribed specific (albeit legally unenforceable) responsibilities, such as taking 'some personal responsibility' for one's health, to 'follow the course of treatment' agreed upon, and 'participate in important public health programmes such as vaccination' (p.9). There is a tension within this image between the 'right to be involved in discussions and decisions about your health care, and to be given information to enable you to do this' (p.7) and the mere 'pledge' that the NHS makes:

> to offer you easily accessible information to enable you to participate fully in your own health care decisions and to support you in making choices. This will include information on the quality of clinical services where there is robust and accurate information available. (p.7)

Describing the provision of information as a pledge seems to imply that the NHS will strive to provide it but not necessarily succeed in doing so – and, as such, is seemingly at odds with the 'right to information'. This highlights a problem in any commitment to enabling participation in health care decision-making, and is, indeed, one that reaches back to the notion of informed consent. If the patient-citizen is to be expected to make a decision that goes beyond the mere expression of a personal whim – that is if they are expected to make a reasonable decision, then they require appropriate information. However, without the appropriate background knowledge in medical science and statistics, the information that the non-specialist can assimilate and critically reflect upon is limited. The pledge perhaps implicitly acknowledges this, reasserting a limited form of professional paternalism in the face of public ignorance. This has perhaps most clearly been manifest in the public response to supposed links between autism and MMR vaccines. The exhortation to the patient-citizen to participate in vaccination programmes can be seen as a rather weak response to that crisis. Such an exhortation avoids the more fundamental problem that encouraging participation in debates over health care, at whatever level, is ineffectual, and, indeed, counter-productive, without a clear articulation of both the nature of professional expertise and the point at which that expertise must trump non-specialist opinions and prejudices. In effect, it is to say that the image of the patient-citizen is, as yet, poorly articulated, and that this poor articulation comes at a cost to the medical professions themselves.

The image of the professional that complements the citizen-patient is similarly paradoxical. The professional is expected to work with integrity, and in accord with all reasonable professional standards. However, more subtly, it is implied that the professional works with a substantial degree of public transparency. While the individual is accountable to their professional body (Department of Health 2009, p.11), the patient's right to information would seem to include, crucially, knowledge of the success and efficiency of medical units (and thus the data being published in 'league tables'). This picks up an important development within the experience of the professional, and a consequence of the failure of New Right thinking. As trust in the professions has eroded over the post-war period, public regulation and monitoring of the professions has increased. Paradoxically, the New Right was ultimately unable to rely on the market as a mechanism of regulation in the provision of what had been public services. The self-interest that guides the provision of good in a free market did not, it seems, necessarily result in the public good that its advocates predicted. This, alongside the exploitation of newly available information technologies, led to the proliferation of methods of monitoring the success or efficiency of medical provision. While such monitoring would seek to protect the public, and merely codify what the professional of integrity would do anyway, regulation and performance targets necessarily lead to a crudeness in the articulation of professional practices. The subtlety and flexibility of everyday professional decision-making is in danger of being sacrificed in order to demonstrate accountability and performance according to given criteria. General comparisons take little account of the contextual differences between the units being compared, and in addition tend to be conservative. The professional's expertise is thus further compromised, as initiative and innovation are penalized, and compliance with protocols is rewarded. The professional is thus in danger of being reduced to a mere practitioner.

More fundamentally, one can argue that statistical data on health care provision also blunts the patient's capacity to make informed choices. Precisely because its quantitative nature necessarily abstracts from the complex moral, technical and social context within which particular decisions are made, statistical data over-simplifies issues and encourages a crude quantitative thinking. Paradoxically, the 'easily accessible information' pledged by the NHS may be counter-productive. The ease of access and assimilation comes at the cost of contextual detail, and the demand to engage in a critical and thoughtful understanding. The patient is thus at once deprived of the qualitative information that is relevant to making genuinely informed choices about health care, and, precisely because alternative forms of data are unavailable, is discouraged from taking a more appropriately critical stance towards the decisions they are required to make. They are, one can argue, thereby thrown back onto making the very consumerist preferences that greater information should allow them to avoid.

There is, it can be suggested, a fundamental confusion at the centre of the relationship between the professional and the citizen-patient. At one level, one can argue that it is perfectly correct and proper that there should be a dialogue between the professional and the patient (and, indeed, general public) on values. There is nothing unreasonable in a patient rejecting a treatment, or even the manner of treatment, on the grounds that it violates their moral sensibilities. In addition, it is highly desirable that the patient has as much technical information as they can cope with, in order that they can make reasonable choices about their own health care, and take responsibility for their health. The confusion occurs if it is then assumed, more or less tacitly, that the patient can legitimately approach matters of scientific evidence with the same attitude that they approach values. In effect, one has to ask what is a reasonable decision on the part of the patient, and – to take the measles, mumps and rubella (MMR) vaccines again as a case in point – whether the patient-citizen has a right to refuse a treatment when there is no good scientific evidence of harm or risk? The conception of the citizen-patient currently avoids this problem, and thus, one can argue, illegitimately undermines the genuine expertise and authority of the professional.

CONCLUSION

The above narrative has sought, more or less explicitly throughout, to address three issues: the changes to the relationships between the professional, the patient and the State; the patient's experience of illness and disease; and, finally, the growing suspicion of the legitimacy of the professional's power. With regard to the last of these, it is evident that professional power has come under increasing attack, and from diverse quarters, through the post-war period. Some of this attack has been well grounded, and the professions have responded responsibly and self-critically to it. However, there have been dangers in these attacks, not least in the implications that they have had for the understanding of the patient. One can suggest that a failure on the part of policymakers adequately to think through either the technical expertise of the professional, or the nature of their moral integrity, has led to autonomy being attributed all too readily to the patient, not least in the New Right articulation of the patient as consumer. This failure adequately to distinguish technical and moral expertise betrays the patient, and crucially does so as the experience of illness and its treatment becomes more complex and daunting to the non-specialist. Although not arguing that a return to a naïve trust in professional expertise is desirable, one can suggest that, at the very least, the grounds of mistrust need to be critically examined as much as do the grounds of trust. The story told above, of the defensiveness of the professions in the face of criticism, now demands a more positive and self-assertive turn.

REFERENCES

Abel-Smith, B. and Townsend, P. (1965) *The Poor and the Poorest: A New Analysis of the Ministry of Labour's 'Family Expenditure Surveys' of 1953–54 and 1960.* London: Bell.

Beauchamp, T.L. and Childress, J.F. (1979) *Principles of Biomedical Ethics* (1st edn). New York: Oxford University Press.

Beveridge, W. (1942) *Social Insurance and Allied Services.* London: HM Stationery Office.

Black, D., Morris, J., Smith, C. and Townsend, P. (1980) *Inequalities in Health: Report of a Research Working Group.* London: Department of Health and Social Security.

Bowling, A. (1993) *What People Say about Prioritising Health Services.* London: King's Fund Centre.

Bowling, A. (1997) *Measuring Health: A Review of Quality of Life Measurement Scales* (2nd edn). Buckingham: Open University Press.

Campbell, A.V. (1995) 'Defining core health services: the New Zealand experience.' *Bioethics 9,* 3/4, 252–258.

Department of Health (1997) *The New NHS.* London: Department of Health.

Department of Health (2001) *The Expert Patient: A New Approach to Chronic Disease Management for the 21st Century.* London: Department of Health.

Department of Health (2009) *The NHS Constitution*. London: Department of Health.

Fink, J. (2005) 'Welfare, Poverty and Social Inequalities.' In P. Addison and H. Jones (eds) *A Companion to Contemporary Britain 1939–2000*. Oxford: Blackwell.

Foucault, M. (1973) *The Birth of the Clinic: An Archaeology of Medical Perception*. London: Tavistock Publications.

Frank, A. (1997) *The Wounded Storyteller: Illness, Body and Ethics*. Chicago, IL: Chicago University Press.

Freidson, E. (1970) *The Profession of Medicine*. New York: Mead and Company.

Giddens, A. (1998) *The Third Way: The Renewal of Social Democracy*. Malden, MA: Polity Press.

Graham, H. (2001) 'The Challenge of Health Inequalities.' In H. Graham (ed.) *Understanding Health Inequalities*. Buckingham: Open University Press.

Hughes, E.C. (1958) *Men and Their Work*. Glencoe, IL: Free Press.

Hunt, S.M., McEwen, J. and McKenna, S. (1986) *Measuring Health Status*. London: Croom Helm.

Ilich, I. (1976) *Limits to Medicine: Medical Nemesis, the Expropriation of Health*. London: Boyars.

Kirk, P. (1993) 'The Oregon Experience.' In M. Turnbridge (ed.) *Rationing of Health Care in Medicine*. London: Royal College of Physicians.

Lowe, R. (2004) *The Welfare State in Britain since 1945*. Basingstoke: Macmillan.

Millerson, G. (1964) *The Qualifying Associations*. London: Routledge and Kegan Paul.

Mohan, J. (2002) *Planning, Markets and Hospitals*. London: Routledge.

Nozick, R. (1974) *Anarchy, State and Utopia*. Oxford: Blackwell.

Oakley, A. (1981) *From Here to Maternity: Becoming a Mother*. Harmondsworth: Penguin.

Parsons, T. (1949) *Essays in Sociological Theory*. New York: Free Press.

Parsons, T. (1951) *The Social System*. New York: Free Press.

Rowntree, B.S. and Lavers, G.R. (1951) *Poverty and the Welfare State: A Third Social Survey of York Dealing Only with Economic Questions*. London: Longmans.

Seedhouse, D. (1986) *Health: The Foundations for Achievement*. Chichester: Wiley.

Spicker, S.F. (1995) 'Going Off the Dole: A Prudential and Ethical Critique of the "Healthfare" State.' In D. Seedhouse (ed.) *Reforming Health Care: The Philosophy and Practice of International Health Reform*. London: John Wiley.

Townsend, P. (1979) *Poverty in the United Kingdom: A Survey of Household Resources and Standards of Living*. Harmondsworth: Penguin.

Chapter 3

Contesting Narratives: Medical Professional Identity Formation amidst Changing Values

Lynn V. Monrouxe and Kieran Sweeney

INTRODUCTION

In order to become successful professionals, those training in a profession must internalize an appropriate professional identity. Key elements of this identity are the values associated with the profession, and, inevitably, some of these associated values will differ from trainees' personally held values. Therefore, in some cases, idealized notions of what it is to be part of that profession may cause internal conflicts in the face of real experience. This is even more likely to occur when professions are undergoing a process of change. Previous work by sociologists and anthropologists on the process of such adaptation to professional values has concentrated on collecting data by direct observation and talking to individuals as they progress through training in areas such as medicine, law and social welfare (Becker *et al.* 1961; Costello 2005; Sinclair 1997). In this chapter, however, we focus on personal incident narratives (PINs) of medical students as they progress through medical school, using data collected by solicited audio diaries. We argue that the careful analysis of these narratives clearly demonstrates how values are created and interpreted in an ongoing and dynamic process of storytelling as individuals struggle to make sense of personal experiences amidst a backdrop of culturally defined narratives of what it is to be a doctor. Here we consider the patterns of social and cognitive processes that help co-create the professional identity of a doctor in a rapidly changing world. This exploration is important, we argue, for reasons that have already been mentioned in earlier chapters.

Society is redefining its relationship to medicine and the medical profession (Irvine 2001). Among the many strands that come together in this revised relationship, the egregious failures of a small number of high-profile cases – for example, Dr Harold Shipman in the UK and Dr Graeme Reeves in Australia – have had a disproportionate influence. The historical status of the doctor is changing irrevocably. Doctors are much less privileged now: they are subject to much greater clinical scrutiny (through the powerful new regulatory bodies such as the Healthcare Commission in the UK) and, when suspected of transgressing agreed professional boundaries are exposed to a much less supine General Medical Council (General Medical Council 2001). The robustness of the medical model itself, upon which so much of the spectacular success of Western biomedicine is predicated, is being re-examined. The conventional view is that the fruits of the Western biomedical model have been of inestimable value to mankind: therapeutically, more can be done now, for more people, more of the time. However, within the profession itself, there is increasing awareness of the importance of the person-as-practitioner – not simply the clinician as professional (Dixon and Sweeney 2000). The work of Michael Polanyi is relevant here (see Polanyi 1958). Having originally gained doctoral degrees in both medicine and physical science, he went on to become Professor of Social Sciences in post-war Manchester. Central to his thinking was the concept of 'tacit knowledge' and its contribution to the generation of new understandings and social and scientific discovery. Emphasis is therefore laid on the importance of personal reflection for the practitioner, in our case the doctor. Starting from the notion of doctor-as-person, we decided to explore those interior experiences, expressed as stories, that help develop medical students into emerging doctors. However, before illustrating the potential of careful analysis of such stories, we will start by setting out in more detail the concepts and theoretical assumptions underpinning our approach.

PROFESSIONAL IDENTITY FORMATION

As discussed above, we argue that professional roles are objectively defined (and redefined) by society. Professional identities are then asserted and claimed through a continual rehearsal of the role until it is converted into a new sense of self – a 'master identity'. Thus the possession of knowledge and skills is a necessary but not sufficient component for professional success: one must also be successful in adopting a professional master identity. It follows that changes in (a) societal expectations of what it is to be a professional and (b) in the education of professionals and in the nature of professional practice will affect how professionals see themselves, i.e. who they think they are in terms of their own attitudes, values, and ethical practice and their view of their broader role in society.

Furthermore, as part of the rehearsal of the role, identities are constructed in and through talk: how we interpret our actions and events, both to ourselves and to others, communicates how we want to be known (Schiffrin 1996). When we narrate stories about events in our lives, we interpret the past in order to present our preferred identities both to ourselves and others. It is therefore possible to gain an understanding of the process of adoption (or rejection) of a master identity through an analysis of individuals' stories over time. Indeed, within any story we can find both explicit (contextual, political, social and cultural discourses)[1] and implicit narratives (taken-for-granted storylines from popular culture) that can be internalized as a social representation of the world and that are developed through our social actions (Moscovici 1988). It is to this idea of narrative that we now turn.

Narrative identity

Stories matter. They enable us to make sense of the world. As we go through everyday life, something happens to us (an event). We then tell others about the something-that-has-happened by way of a story. In telling this story we impose a structure, including the identification of a beginning–middle–end temporal sequence, which was not present in the lived experience but which is considered necessary for us to 'make sense' of that lived experience both to ourselves and to others (Ricoeur 1992). Ultimately, our own narratives are constructions that

---

1   Discourses are ways in which our knowledge of society and the roles people play in society are
     acted out in everyday talk.

help us make sense of who we were, who we are and who we might be. Furthermore, we draw upon cultural plotlines as we construct narratives about ourselves and the world. These discourses can be conceived as social representations that both influence and constitute social practices (Howarth 2006).[2]

Representations and action

Having touched on the notion that the process of a narrative identity entails representations that inform action, we would now like to explain briefly what we mean by this. Although it's not always acknowledged (researchers working with the field of narrative enquiry and those working within the domain of social representation are not one and the same) we believe that there are links between the two perspectives, and these can be traced back to studies of collective representations and the role of social processes in memory. In fact, Moscovici (1988) brought these ideas together in his 'social representation theory', in which he proposed that social representations are created and re-created through interactions and that this is how individuals come to understand everyday concepts (including values). According to this perspective, rather than being static, cognitive schemas, social representations are defined as being active and dynamic 'existing only in the relational encounter, the in-between space we create in dialogue and negotiation with others' (Howarth 2006, p.68). In other words, our thoughts are not isolated from the social and so we continually construct and co-construct a framework of shared references – social representations – that define how we think about ourselves and about the world.

However, in addition to the notion of social representations existing in a relational encounter with an audience, Mead links the social and individual when he argues that the most important audience is ourselves:

> There is a field, a sort of inner forum, in which we are the only spectators and the only actors. In that field each one of us confers with himself. He asks and answers questions. He develops his ideas and arranges and organises those ideas

---

2   'A backdrop of cultural expectations about a typical course of action; our identities as social beings emerge as we construct our own individual experiences as a way to position ourselves in relation to social and cultural expectations' (Schiffrin 1996, p.170).

as he might do in conversation with somebody else. (Mead
1936, p.401)

Considering the role of the self in this process and turning to the domain
of cognitive science, we can add the following related principles of
connectionism: 'Thought is structured through neural activity. Language
is inextricable from thought and experience' (Feldman 2008, p.3).

Through these two principles, the understanding of the inner
forum and the patterning of social interaction, we argue that we can
comprehend how the social and psychological are part of each other and
together bring about the development of the self. Ultimately, we believe
that representations are dynamically intertwined through both social
and cognitive processes, and it is through the patterning of this dynamic
intertwining that change occurs.

UNDERSTANDING TRANSITIONS IN PROFESSIONAL IDENTITY TRANSFORMATION

In October 2005 we began a longitudinal research study to investigate
17 medical students' professional-identity formation over time. Our aim
was to understand how individuals entering medical education narrated
their developing identities as medical students of today and doctors of
tomorrow, through the spontaneous stories they related over time. The
solicited audio-diary was the primary means of data collection since
we wanted participants to decide for themselves what to tell us. Thus,
students were given a Dictaphone and asked to record a message for
the study whenever they wished. Our request was simple: 'Please tell us
a story about something that has happened to you since the last time
you left a message and how it has affected the way you think about
yourself now and your future role as a doctor.' This method was used
to gather students' stories of particular events that held meaning for
them personally, with minimal influence from the researcher in order
to understand how students constructed their developing identity as
doctors of tomorrow (Monrouxe 2009).

This work is ongoing, and our analyses to date consider the first
18 months of the study. A total of 255 diary entries were received (a diary
entry comprises one or more recording made in a single 24-hour period),
which comprised 408 separate recordings (from 20 seconds, up to 13:57).
Students recorded their diary entry, then emailed it to the first author.

As we listened to these recordings, we were continually amazed by the depth of reflection (and at times, emotion) displayed in the diverse events recounted by the students as they began to construct their own developing professional narratives.

While there were some differences, there were also many commonalities in terms of what participants talked about. For example, they discussed issues of personal change, recounting stories of incidents during which their own embodied worldview was exposed to and compared with other, sometimes incompatible, worldviews. Thus some narratives revealed the evolution of their own attitudes and values, while others suggested the potential for clinging to prior values. Some messages explored the tensions that participants felt when they found themselves in situations involving conflicting social roles, identities and/or needs, while others demonstrated when participants' different identities became synchronized. Further stories recounted ways in which participants' relationships with bodies, their own and those of others, were affected during the early months of medical training.

Thus a number of key master narratives were apparent, together with others that appeared to contest them. Such contesting narratives appeared to be echoes of discourses frequently found within the current culture of a modern medical school. These included the 'Informed Servant' narrative whereby the doctor acts predominantly as expert resource – rather than expert professional – setting out the alternative therapeutic strategies, having initially framed the patient's dilemma. This contests the dominant 'Certainty of Medicine' narrative, frequently found in clinical environments, in which biomedical knowledge is privileged above all other types of knowing. It also contests the 'Healing Doctor' narrative whereby the role of the doctor is to heal the sick. The 'Uncertainty of Medicine' narrative also contests the 'Certainty of Medicine' narrative and reflects the way in which these students, the doctors of tomorrow, are being educated. This narrative is interesting as a reflection of society's changing attitudes about the role of medicine and doctors. As noted in previous chapters, commentators have claimed that attitudes are moving from deferential acceptance to active consumer-based critique. The 'Uncertainty' narrative in the students' stories illustrates their exploration of the epistemological basis informing and supporting the predominant 'Certainty of Medicine' theme and is distinguished from the 'Informed Servant' narrative, which depicts and explores the role of doctoring.

What we find particularly interesting and relevant are the diary entries in which the participants narrated the tensions they experienced between dominant and contesting narratives, during which they attempted to make sense of their identities as doctors of tomorrow. At times, this sense-making process was emotionally charged, appearing to cause sometimes painful and frustrating internal conflict within participants as they negotiated their way through their previously held notions of what it is to be a doctor and the events that unfolded during their own experiences that challenged those ideals and values. It is to one of these narratives that we will now turn.

PAUL'S NARRATIVE

Paul was 21 and at the beginning of his second year at medical school. His recording lasted 29 minutes and 41 seconds and comprised a number of small stories within this longer narrative. We present an edited version of the longer narrative. The narrative contains the core structure of a narrative identified by Labov and Waletzky (1967) and includes the following elements:

- Abstract (general overview of the story)
- Orientation (whereby the listener is introduced to key players and settings of the story)
- Complicating Action (essentially, what happened)
- Evaluation of what happened

We also identify the 'signifying sentence', which alerts the listener that the narrator is about to disclose a Complicating Action. While the event narrated in the story (the Complicating Action) is an important aspect of the shaping of identities, more crucial in this development is the sense-making process revealed in the Evaluation. Since space does not permit a detailed analysis, our focus in the following discussion will be on key aspects of this narrative that are highly revealing with respect to Paul's evolving identity as a doctor.

ABSTRACT[3]

1. Okay hello-I thought I'd just say something about the placement that we had last
2. week...Yes I saw loads of different cases-

SIGNIFYING SENTENCE

3. I mean there was nothing-at that point there was nothing like-erm <u>hugely</u> different-...

ORIENTATION

4. and then the GP came back up again and got me and he basically said that-that I could
5. go with him to-on his visits-cause he had about two patients outside the GP clinic
6. which obviously required him to go see them (0.5) so I obviously said yes to that and
7. off we went to a-to a nursing home...and then we obviously met-met the patient-well-I
8. got to know the environment where his patients were staying and it's basically just a
9. converted house-just tiny little hallways going to this room-going to that room-and it
10. was just erm-full of elderly people obviously because it was a nursing home-

COMPLICATING ACTION

11. and one of the particular patients was actually in a bed and she wasn't looking very
12. healthy at all-and she wasn't moving much she had a mouth wide open-she was
13. really-looked really skinny and-kind of-really in a bad shape basically-and

ORIENTATION

14. apparently she been throwing up blood all morning cause she had a gastric ulcers and
15. also she was insulin-dependent-she was diabetic-and it basically-I think she had
16. dementia as well-and she was basically bedbound the last four days-throwing up blood

---

3   Transcript notations: <u>Underlined</u> = emphasized; Hyphen-at-end-= running on speech; ((...)) = inaudible speech; (.) = micropause; (1.5) = pause to nearest half second; ... = omitted speech; numbers on the left identify line numbers for ease of cross referencing.

17. and really not in good shape and the doctor was basically telling me all of this

COMPLICATING ACTION

18. and I was wondering how-how would you treat someone in this condition-and he was

19. saying 'well, you obviously-if someone's throwing up blood and they've got-they've got

20. gastric ulcers who had obviously taken into hospital and go into surgery and have it

21. operated on' but this-this woman-this elderly woman was obviously-I think she was 80-

22. 85-and she was basically in no state to go to hospital and the success-the criteria to have

23. that kind of surgery-you know-they have to have some kind of erm-good health before

24. they go in-so they can survive the operation-and obviously that was an issue and that

25. basically meant she wasn't going to be sent to the hospital because she would have the

26. operation and then stay bedbound for another three-three months and obviously-it doesn't

27. add to her quality of life-well he thought it wouldn't add to her quality of life-so then

SIGNIFYING SENTENCE

28. obviously I was wondering what he was going to get up to-er-what he was getting at-

COMPLICATING ACTION

29. and he was actually saying that 'you can't take them to hospital-er-can't take her to

30. hospital because she can't get treated on and you can't-you can't leave her in bed all the

31. time because there's no quality of life' and so at that point I was really-'so what is he

32. saying? is he saying he's just going to let her pass away?' and it turns out he-he was

33. saying that the patient needs to-the relatives need to come in and they obviously had a

34. chat with the doctor already and he decided that they would put a morphine driver-which

35. is basically a small drip of morphine-not a drip-sorry-a kind of a catheter into-into one

36. of the veins-just erm delivering a bit of morphine every now and then just to ease the

37. pain-cause obviously she might be in great pain from the gastric ulcers that she had-

38. but once that is in it's basically erm-making her bedbound and she wouldn't be able to

39. move again-she wouldn't have as much pain-she wouldn't be in a lot of pain-which

40. is obviously a <u>good</u> thing but she would have no quality of life-she's obviously insulin-

41. dependent-so in order to survive she also needs to have these insulin shots to control her

42. blood glucose-blood sugar-erm-and basically what the doctor was saying was once the

43. screwdriver was in-we-er-we stop treatment-er so stop any nutritional like vitamins and

44. supplements-and stop the insulin treatment and basically that would-that would put her-

45. because actually she's erm-kind of has these really high peaks of glucose and can't

46. control it because she's insulin dependent-so basically it means she would go into a coma

47. because there was so much glucose in her blood-this-by having the morphine driver

48. it means she could peacefully get into this coma and once she is in a coma if-without

49. treatment should obviously passed away in her sleep-and this is what he was telling me-

EVALUATION

50. and I was-I was almost half shocked-and I still am in a way that-I don't-I wasn't sure

51. what I expected-I wasn't sure what they did in this kind of situation-obviously this is

52. what they do-they-they put the morphine driver and allow her to go into a coma and

53. have a peaceful death-cause-the quality of life without that would-it's just deteriorating

54. and it's bad and the relatives have approved and...he had to take that decision-basically

55. saying that he's kind of sure that there is no hidden interest like that and it will probably
56. be the best for the patient so-he was acting in the patient's best interest which is what
57. he was saying (0.5) so at that point-you know I was still slightly shocked

COMPLICATING ACTION
58. and also he went on to say-to say the nurses were viewing-were doing their normal
59. duties and then suddenly this patient starts to throw up a lot of blood and is really-seems
60. to be in a lot of pain-and then increase the morphine-the morphine dosage which
61. essentially-what he was saying would actually-would actually kill her and put her into a
62. respiratory failure and basically kill her-you know because the morphine would just-
63. not allow her to do anything-and then she would obviously die-

EVALUATION
64. and so for me that's almost like assisted suicide or euthanasia if you like-and yet still
65. quite shocked at the fact that he-that the doctor would recommend that-it was obviously
66. in the patient's best interest but I'm still not quite sure (0.5) anyway-that was-yeah-that
67. was interesting to see how-how the doctor deals with that kind of situation-but obviously
68. it was fairly-fairly sad really and I almost was thinking that's probably one of the aspects
69. of the job that I wouldn't actually enjoy in-erm you know in the future-and so-
70. yeah it was still-still a bit of a shock

ORIENTATIONS (TO NEXT STORY)
71. and with that basically we moved on-we went on to the next patient they had-and yeah-
72. she-she turned out to be an elderly woman again...

EVALUATION (OF ENTIRE NARRATIVE)
73. yeah-so that visit to the nursing home ended up being a fairly-ended up on a good note

74. basically-I learnt a lot about-erm-about what you do and when someone is just almost-

75. almost passing away and how to deal with it and-it's slightly shocking obviously-

(RETURN TO COMPLICATING ACTION OF FIRST STORY)

76. like I said-yeah-'it's a fact of life' that's what the doctor was saying-and 'this is just the

77. best for the patient'

EVALUATION

78. -which is obviously what the General Medical Council tells us we should do is-always

79. act in the patient's best interest-so yeah-

COMMENTARY ON PAUL'S NARRATIVE

Paul's narrative involves his encounter with an 85-year-old, insulin-dependent woman with dementia who is suffering gastrointestinal bleeding. He narrates the doctor's dilemma as being that both surgeons and anaesthetists would probably decline to treat her and, even if they agreed to, it is likely that she would die during the procedure. However, if not offered these interventions, she will die anyway. The aspect of good clinical practice brought to bear in these situations is how to proceed in a compassionate, technically appropriate and acceptable manner – 'acceptable' here implying acceptable in professional terms and also in the eyes of the family. Paul's narrative includes an indication of his own pre-understandings of the world, as he tries to make sense of these events. What is interesting about this excerpt is that we can see how this developing professional struggles with who he was, who he is now, and who he may become professionally in light of this experience. This struggle is articulated through Paul's rhetorical use of the word 'shock' (lines 50, 57, 65, 70 and 75), as he describes his reaction to the event.

Of further interest is the way in which Paul configures time, the impact that this has on how he comes to terms with this 'shocking' event, and how he incorporates this understanding within his evolving identity as a doctor. From the beginning of his longer narrative, Paul indicates that he has something important to talk about in his diary entry, but that this would not be revealed immediately ('I mean there was nothing-at that point there was nothing...' see line 3, which comes

1 min 16 sec into the recording). Instead, Paul chooses to locate this critical incident towards the middle of his longer story about the day's experiences ('we obviously met the patient...' line 7, 8 min 24 sec into the recording). Furthermore, when he introduces this formative event, he does so in an almost casual storytelling manner, as he orients the listener to the nursing home setting (line 7). Indeed, the only telling point in this narrative orientation indicating that this incident is indeed critical, is his referral to meeting *the* patient, when the nursing home incident he recounts actually involves two patients. The second patient is narrated as being 'unproblematic' – cheerful and smiling despite being bed-bound (not included in the above excerpt) – enabling him to smooth over the troublesome event in his longer narrative of the nursing home visit, as having 'ended up on a good note' (line 73).

The temporal placement of this critical incident within his longer story – putting it in the middle and ensuring a positive ending – is only one way in which Paul configures time in his narrative. He also conflates the time dimension in the process of events. He introduces the graphic description of the patient 'throwing up blood' early on (this exact phrase is used three times in quick succession – lines 14, 16 and 19) and later links this action to an increase in morphine dose during his description of the Complicating Action of giving morphine (line 59). However, in reality this decision is nuanced, and is usually anticipated and specifically allowed for in the technically demanding writing of the 24-hour prescription of the diamorphine (note, not morphine) dose.

In addition to considering temporal aspects of this narrative, we are also drawn to the way in which Paul sometimes aligns himself with the GP doctor (and nurses), and other times effectively distances himself through his use of personal pronouns such as 'we', 'I' and 'he'. Thus, Paul begins by aligning himself with the doctor: 'we obviously met-met the patient' (line 7). Later, when he begins to describe the Complicating Action and the rationale behind giving morphine, he initially reports this in a factual manner, which might be interpreted as being Paul's own opinion. Possibly realizing this, he immediately distances himself by attributing the statement to the opinion of the doctor: 'it doesn't add to her quality of life-well he thought it wouldn't add to her quality of life...' (lines 26–27). Furthermore, and by way of distancing himself even further from events, he immediately utters a Signifying Sentence: 'I was wondering what he was going to get up to-er-what he was getting at'. This sentence is key in that it reveals Paul's own concerns that what the doctor proposes is effectively euthanasia/assisted suicide – revealed later – and his struggle with accepting what he sees as his new role as a doctor – to carry this out.

Paul then describes his understanding of the doctor's dilemma: 'you can't take them to hospital…because she can't get treated…you can't leave her in bed all the time because there's no quality of life' (lines 29–31). This aspect of Paul's narrative is interesting, as his beliefs about this dilemma and the role of a doctor are revealed through his use of the impersonal 'you' within reported speech attributed to the GP (Holt and Clift 2007). Impersonal 'you' marks an informal, conversational speech style and is sometimes employed to communicate a generally admitted 'truth', when speakers want their audience to share their views (Kitagawa and Lehrer 1990). In this context, 'you' refers to doctors in general – and this includes Paul, who is training to be a doctor, as Paul situated it within the reported talk of the GP to himself. Furthermore, this use of the referential 'you' is followed by verbs of obligation (three times Paul reports the doctor as saying 'you can't'), thereby signalling the power and authority of the speaker (the doctor) to the audience (Paul). So Paul is telling us here that, as a doctor he will be faced with this dilemma, that these are the facts as conveyed by a figure of authority, and that it is a quality of life issue.

However, Paul's sense-making process as he narrates this event demonstrates a readiness to accept the situation as he carefully constructs his narrative around concepts of good (line 40) and bad (line 54) within this quality of life matter (lines 27, 31, 40 and 53), leaving it until relatively late in the narrative to voice his own personal concerns that this may be 'almost like assisted suicide or euthanasia' (line 64). Furthermore, we can see that while Paul narrates the events, and constructs the rationale for these events around the notion of goodness and quality of life issues, he is able to associate himself with this community of practice through the use of the exclusive pronoun 'we' (here, meaning those in the medical profession, specifically doctors and nurses): 'we-er-we stop treatment' (line 43). However, as he enters a sequential evaluative stage in this narrative he immediately introduces his own anxiety surrounding the unfolding events, and confessing to feeling shocked, he then switches to using the distancing pronoun 'they' as he tries to make sense of what 'doctors do' in this kind of situation: 'I wasn't sure what they did in this kind of situation-this is obviously what they do-they-they put in the morphine driver…' (lines 51–52).

Through these notions of good and bad within a quality of life issue, and the process of aligning himself with the good and distancing himself from the bad, Paul is able to accept the unacceptable as it is for the benefit of the patient. Thus he begins the process of adopting this aspect of 'what you do' as doctor in such situations (line 74). Finally, Paul briefly returns to the Complicating Action, narrating solely within the reported speech of the doctor, summarizing events as being the only course of action: "'it's a fact of life" that's what the doctor was saying- and "this is just the best for the patient"' (lines 76–77). He further underscores this concept of acting in the patient's best interest in his final evaluation of the event by appealing to General Medical Council guidelines (line 79).

So, it seems that Paul's configuration of time enables him to resolve his own dilemma between his representation of the role of a doctor – doctors save lives and don't kill people – which is at odds with his experience: this doctor is going to kill someone (interpreted through his representations of the concept of euthanasia). First, Paul's configuration of time makes the story more acceptable to himself (and others) as he constructs a beginning, middle and end – including a successful resolution to his day. This resolution enables Paul to accept 'shocking' events as being part of a longer and more positively focused story of what it is to be a doctor. Second, by conflating time in his description of critical events, he has effectively dramatized those events to construct a strong rationale for giving morphine to the patient. This conflation of time therefore enables him to accept what he would once have not accepted as he defers to the authority of the doctor and society, saying that this would contribute to a good death, would reduce her pain, and would, generally, be in her best interests. Thus we see the development of a shift in Paul's narrative identity – that he's now joining a community of people who do not save lives, but a community of people who manage death.

CONCLUSIONS
Implications for the profession
The argument in this chapter proposes that an individual's attitudes develop as social representations, continuously co-created through social interaction, from which emerges a framework of shared references helping us to make sense of our world. If one accepts, from connectionism,

that representations are states of cognitive activation reflecting our interactions with the world, one can discern a further link between those attitudes as representations, and Ricoeur's (1992) perspective on identity formation. For the authors, this presents us with the challenge of exploring narratives: those texts, symbols and signs – exchanged, told and re-told in a continuing sense-making pattern – from which emerges the person one has come to be. Why should this be important for clinicians and medical educators?

First, doctors are people too. They are not, as a function of their medical training, immunized from the fears, prejudices, joys and disappointments of the human predicament. Doctors are not passive recipients of, nor simple conduits for, clinical evidence. They conduct inner consultations with evidence, and show themselves to be vulnerable to both the 'availability heuristic' (we recall mainly those events that are more easily recalled), and the 'chagrin factor' (doctors tend to avoid actions that cause them hassle). Therefore the profession needs urgently to theorize about the ways in which the doctor-as-person is intertwined with the doctor-as-clinician. Conventionally, the process of elaborating therapeutic advice in a consultation is thought to be predicated on a neutral, objective assessment of evidence relating to the presenting clinical problem, objectively abstracted from the patient's story. But thinking and feeling are indivisible: we personally participate in every act of comprehension we make (Polanyi 1958). No act of knowing can be achieved without involving passion. Here we have explored the interior, intra-personal activities that form the patterns by which a person-doctor comes to be that person-doctor. How that person forms their attitudes, what types of knowledge that person privileges, and how that person moulds their attitudes, become important areas to clarify and understand. For clinical educators, this underlines the importance of teasing out the distinctions between the explicit and tacit/hidden curricula in medical schools, and encouraging students to articulate any tensions they may experience as they internalize their professional identity, which may be in conflict with their own identity.

The second reason supporting the authors' perspective in this chapter relates to the role of science in Western biomedicine. Advances in clinical science, predicated on the philosophy of positivism, and supported by the principles of probability statistics, have been of huge benefit to mankind. But science does not do the work of medicine – doctors (people) do. When deciding what to do for a patient, doctors are guided by two levels of significance: statistical (from probability theory) and clinical (evidence-based medicine). However, if we elevate the importance of the doctor as person, and accept that, in an exchange with a patient both parties are subtly moulding and being moulded, then we are forced to consider what has been called a 'third dimension', that of personal significance.

This becomes more relevant in contemporary clinical practice, where advances in therapy mean doctors can do more, for more people, more of the time. For the next generation of doctors, perhaps the most demanding clinical question will be, 'When is enough, enough?', and the most demanding clinical dilemma will be when to discontinue treatment. These decisions become acutely relevant in the very old patient, where preventing death from one cause simply increases the chances of death by another. These decisions are arrived at after lengthy discussions, usually with the patient, the patient's family and the clinician in a triad, and are the emergent property of these interactions.

The analysis of these extremely common and important clinical discussions needs to have a sound theoretical basis, needs to be clearly understood before they can be taught, and needs to be constantly revised as scientific knowledge advances. These discussions will become more complex as molecular medicine becomes more mainstream, and, as society redefines its relationship with doctors – their role being as expert adviser, informing the patient of options. Increasingly, people will live longer in chronic illness, with often two or more debilitating medical conditions co-existing. Paradoxically, this state will be both caused by, and supported by, advances in medical science.

How a doctor conceptualizes suffering, deals with it personally, and can handle it in the therapeutic encounter, all become important activities to understand, and we argue that their theoretical basis lies in the propositions we have outlined here. Clearly, the notion of suffering will be increasingly important in medical student education, as the emerging doctor is prepared for life in the real world.

We all have 'our view from somewhere' (Polkinghorne 2001). Doctors, we argue, develop their 'view from somewhere' continuously, emergently, as a function of the interaction with others, through the patterned intertwining of cognitive and social processes. These patterns can be discerned in the narratives people recount, in a continuing process of sense-making. Research that can systematically analyse such insights into the developments of one's identity can help us understand the processes involved, and, in turn, help us develop educational strategies to legitimize reflective practice and narrative sensitivity as the centre of medical education.

ACKNOWLEDGEMENTS

We would like to thank the participants of our research for sharing their stories with us and especially to 'Paul' for allowing us to reproduce his narrative here. We would also like to thank the Nuffield Foundation and Support for Science for their grants, which helped in funding this project.

RESPONSE
Brian Hurwitz

I think the work the authors report here is quite pioneering in its field, but I found the chapter a little scary! It seeks to elucidate some of the processes by which medical students develop professional medical identities, a murky and important area to know more about. Its centrepiece is an in-depth analysis of an account by a second-year student, Paul, chosen from 255 audio-recordings made by medical students responding to a research request to 'Tell us a story about something that has happened to you…and how it has affected the way you think about yourself now and your future role as a doctor.' Two aspects of the chapter scare me – perhaps they are best described as 'emphases' – and these are interrelated:

- First, the authors conceptualize professionalism as predominantly a matter of self-image – 'how professionals see themselves: who they think they are in terms of their own attitudes, values, ethical practice and in terms of their broader role in society' – at the expense of closer consideration of the power relations embodied by professional formations in society. The result is that the authors' work could be seen as buttressing role-modelling (albeit with a stronger self-conscious approach to such modelling) as the means for learning about professional medical identity.

- Second, whilst they rightly pay attention to 'the notion of the doctor-as-person', the chapter offers surprisingly little focus on the embodied personhood of patients.

The effect of both of these emphases is to tilt the argument towards analysis that pivots around medical self-awareness, professional activities, discourse and justification, rather than around how professional identity might emerge from the balance of power between different groupings and the perspectives of those groups in society.

The authors clearly view professional identity as something co-created by social and cognitive processes, and they agree with Irvine (2001) that society is redefining its relationship to medicine and the medical profession. But their claim that certain 'egregious failures of a small number of high-profile cases, such as Dr Harold Shipman in the UK...have had a disproportionate influence' on loss of public trust in the professional status of doctors and their institutions is a formulation that worries me. There are several other notable examples in the UK illustrating problems with some of the profession's institutions and the poor manner in which its practitioners and officers have operated certain health care arrangements and regulations over a long period (30 years), some of which led to civil investigations. Examples include:

- information withheld from parents about high mortality rates from paediatric cardiac-switch operations at Bristol Royal Infirmary (Kennedy 2001)

- retention of organs and tissues from post-mortems without permission over many decades across the UK (Marshall 2007; The Redfern Inquiry 2007)

- insufficient checks on doctors referred to the General Medical Council for Professional Misconduct (Department of Health 2000)

- practitioners struck off medical registers abroad wrongly allowed to practise in the UK

- a rickety NHS complaints system.

The subsequent investigations especially criticized the inward-looking and insular culture of medicine, which to some extent patrols the self-identity of the medical profession. Professional attitudes and values have been found to be isolated from those of the public and from society's expectations, expressed, for example, in developments in common law that demand much greater openness and provision of information to patients (see Kennedy 2001; Maclean 2009).

In Foucault's words:

> power and knowledge directly imply one another…there is no power relation without the correlative constitution of a field of knowledge, nor any knowledge that does not presuppose and constitute at the same time power relations. (Foucault 1982, p.27)

The expert, including the medical expert, commands not only a corpus of knowledge, ethics and values but also a set of interests (including self-interests), which express themselves in the figure of the doctor – in the doctor's status in relation to patients, the professional group and society at large. True, many of these relationships are under intense scrutiny at the present time, but not (as might be thought) like never before. In the 'long eighteenth century', the period of 1700–1850, Corfield notes the groundswell of public dissatisfaction with the arrangements for medical care, especially sharply expressed in the work of writers and artists:

> No part of the medical profession escaped censure for greed and callousness. In numerous prints and cartoons, dentists wrenched teeth out brutally, midwives were gross and drink-sodden, physicians fought over dying patients, prescribed unpleasant medicines, and made clandestine love to wives and maidservants. (Corfield 2005, p.57)

That groundswell of dissatisfaction and protest identified many faults in the relationship between doctor and patient, and with provision of health care at the time, and in the nineteenth century resulted in processes of progressive state intervention in licensing and registration of apothecaries and doctors – and later in their education.

Shipman was a GP in Hyde, Greater Manchester, who was convicted in 1998 of 15 murders and of forging a will (Baker 2001; Smith 2005). He was found by two separate enquiries using entirely different methodologies to have unlawfully killed some 215 patients (and likely 30 more), people who were not terminally ill or in pain, and who were not otherwise ill. Many of Shipman's bizarre and divergent practices were detected but were neither properly registered nor investigated. The two investigations, together with the criminal trial of Shipman, revealed systemic and deep failures in many health care and health service systems, not all of which can be put down to abuses by the medical profession. However, many of the systems that failed to detect his activities were operated by members of the profession, sometimes rather poorly, and the few members of the profession who had pointed to its failures and called for their reform had been isolated and ignored over many years (Havard 1960; Hurwitz 2004; Hurwitz 2005; Simpson 1978). Power can also be exercised by silence and inactivity (Baker and Hurwitz 2009).

In their chapter, Monrouxe and Sweeney promise a consideration of identity formation today, in the context of images engendered by occupancy of medical roles created by agencies of medicine, society and the State. 'Iteration' and 'rehearsal' of such social and medical roles generate (in ways that are not specified and are probably unknown) a sense of collective self, a 'master identity' expressed, perhaps, in formal statements of value, such as guidelines and ethical principles, in hierarchical relations and doctor–patient relationships and more informally within local fora, conversations between doctors and others (including medical students). From analysis of medical student audio-recordings (n=255 to date), the authors find certain 'key narratives' concerning identity formation to be 'dominant', 'contesting' and 'in tension' with each other, such as 'the Informed Servant', 'the Certainty of Medicine' and 'Uncertainty of Medicine' narratives (which, they note, are also found both in professional discourses and within inner fora – struggles within the selves of individual professionals and students).

I expected to see these narratives taken up in the analysis of the transcript of Paul's account about 'two patients outside the GP clinic which obviously required him to go and see them'. But instead, Paul's account is presented as a discourse, split up by narrative headings suggested by Labov and Waletzky (1967), and summarized by the authors as follows:

> Paul's narrative involves his encounter with an 85-year-old, insulin-dependent woman with dementia who is suffering gastrointestinal bleeding. He [Paul] narrates the doctor's dilemma as being that both surgeons and anaesthetists would probably decline to treat her and, even if they agreed to, it is likely that she would die during the procedure.

However, if not offered these interventions, she will die anyway. (Monrouxe and Sweeney, p.72)

If this summary accurately represents what Paul was confronting it might not surprise readers that within the excerpt transcript offered Paul expresses 'shock' on five occasions in relation to what he's describing. The authors believe that Paul's shock reveals 'a developing professional struggling with who he was (before becoming a medical student), who he is now, and who he may become professionally in light of this experience'. But is this really the way in which the situation and health care options of this old lady were conceptualized by her GP, and depicted by Paul in his audio-tape? From the data presented, the summary rendering they offer looks 'over interpreted' and based upon a stock view of what a case history stripped of patient identity and embodied individuality 'should' look (and sound) like (Hurwitz 2006).

This old lady, as described here, appears to have no voice. Decisions are being made for her by her health carers in association, we learn, with her relatives. Paramount in the decision-making process is that she should not be in pain (how much pain is she in?), but as readers, we gain no real sense that she has been recognized as a person, albeit sick, dying and perhaps speechless. Who knows her (does the GP know her)?, How long have her carers known her? and What do they know about her? are all questions demanding urgent answers.

Given the potency of this tale in the formation of a medical student's potential identification with a modern professional medical role, this was the second scary element of the chapter for me. I suspect Paul was also scared, perhaps of the power of the profession to make such reductive vignettes, perhaps even more of the possibility that this old lady may be given amounts of opiates that would shorten her life. Both these possibilities are expressions of real power that I would like to have seen more focus on in a chapter about the creation of professional identities.

REFERENCES

Baker, R. (2001) *Harold Shipman's Clinical Practice 1974–1998*. London: Department of Health.

Baker, R. and Hurwitz, B. (2009) 'Intentionally Harmful Violations and Patient Safety: The Example of Harold Shipman.' In B. Hurwitz and A. Sheikh (eds) *Health Care Errors and Patient Safety*. Oxford: BMJ Books, Blackwell Publishing.

Becker, H., Geer, B., Hughes, E. and Strauss, A. (1961) *Boys in White: Student Culture in Medical School*. Chicago, IL,: University of Chicago Press.

Corfield, P.J. (2005) *Power and the Professions in Britain 1700–1850*. London: Routledge.

Costello, C.Y. (2005) *Professional Identity Crisis: Race, Class, Gender and Success at Professional Schools.* Nashville, TN: Vanderbilt University Press.

Department of Health (2000) *An Inquiry into Quality and Practice within the National Health Service arising from the Actions of Rodney Ledward.* London: The Stationery Office.

Dixon, M. and Sweeney, K.G. (2000) *The Human Effect in Medicine: Theory Research and Practice.* Oxford: Radcliffe Press.

Feldman, J.A. (2008) *From Molecule to Metaphor: A Neural Theory of Language.* Cambridge, MA: Massachusetts Institute of Technology Press.

Foucault, M. (1982) *Discipline and Punish.* Harmondsworth: Penguin.

General Medical Council (2001) *Good Medical Practice.* London: General Medical Council.

Havard, J.D. (1960) *The Detection of Secret Homicide.* London: Macmillan.

Holt, E. and Clift, R. (2007) *Reporting Talk: Reported Speech in Interaction.* Cambridge: Cambridge University Press.

Howarth, C. (2006) 'A social representation is not a quiet thing: exploring the critical potential of social representations theory.' *British Journal of Social Psychological Society 45,* 1, 65–86.

Hurwitz, B. (2004) 'Murder most medical, disposal most discreet.' *The Lancet 364,* 38–39.

Hurwitz, B. (2005) 'Many of Shipman's bizarre and divergent practices were detected but were neither properly registered nor investigated [letter].' *British Medical Journal.* Available at http://bmj.bmjjournals.com/cgi/eletters/331/7513/411#114726, accessed on 24 June 2009.

Hurwitz, B. (2006) 'Form and representation in clinical case reports.' *Literature and Medicine 25,* 2, 216–240.

Irvine, D. (2001) 'The changing relationship between the public and the medical profession.' *Journal of the Royal Society of Medicine 94,* 4, 162–169.

Kennedy, I. (chair) (2001) *Learning from Bristol. The Report of the Public Enquiry into Children's Heart Surgery at the Bristol Royal Infirmary 1984–1995.* London: The Stationery Office.

Kitagawa, C. and Lehrer, A. (1990) 'Impersonal uses of personal pronouns.' *Journal of Pragmatics 14,* 5, 739–759.

Labov, W. and Waletzky, J. (1967) 'Narrative analysis.' *Journal of Narrative and Life History 7,* 3–39.

Maclean, M. (2009) 'The Many Advantages and Some Disadvantages of a No-blame Culture Regarding Medical Errors.' In B. Hurwitz and A. Sheikh (eds) *Health Care Errors and Patient Safety.* Oxford: BMJ Books, Blackwell Publishing.

Marshall, T. (2007) *Stolen Hearts.* Nottingham: Critical, Cultural and Communication Press.

Mead, G.H. (1936) *Movement of Thought in the Nineteenth Century.* Chicago, IL: Chicago University Press.

Monrouxe, L.V. (2009) 'Solicited audio diaries in longitudinal narrative research: a view from inside.' *Qualitative Research 9,* 1, 81–103.

Moscovici, S. (1988) 'Notes towards a description of social representations.' *European Journal of Social Psychology 18,* 3, 211–250.

Polanyi, M. (1958) *Personal Knowledge: Towards a Post Critical Philosophy.* Chicago, IL: Chicago University Press.

Polkinghorne, J. (2001) *Faith, Science and Understanding.* New York: Yale University Press.

The Redfern Inquiry into Human Tissue Analysis in UK Nuclear Facilities (2007). Available at www.theredferninquiry.co.uk, accessed on 24 June 2009.

Ricoeur, P. (1992) *Oneself as Another.* Chicago, IL: University of Chicago Press.

Schiffrin, D. (1996) 'Narrative as self-portrait: sociolinguistic constructions of identity.' *Language in Society 25,* 2, 167–203.

Simpson, K. (1978) *Forty Years of Murder.* London: Harrap.

Sinclair, S. (1997) *Making Doctors: an Institutional Apprenticeship.* Oxford: Berg.

Smith, J. (chair) (2005) *Shipman: The Final Report.* Available at www.the-shipman-inquiry.org.uk/finalreport.asp, accessed on 24 June 2009.

Chapter 4

General Practitioners and their Values in a Late Modern World

Roisin Pill

INTRODUCTION

General practice has a key position in the provision of health care under the British National Health Service (NHS), providing free-of-charge primary care to the vast majority of the population. The general practitioner (GP) acts as a gatekeeper and controller of access to a range of expensive hospital specialist services (Calnan and Gabe 1991). However, the NHS has also been described as an institution that is constantly re-inventing itself, like a car that is being re-engineered even while it is roaring round the test track (Ranade 1998).

These comments suggest that a closer examination of the relationship between GPs and the State – their employer – might be particularly illuminating when thinking about professional values in a changing health care context. As noted in Chapter 1, earlier commentators often used the doctor as the epitome of the ideal type of a professional, i.e. someone with a vocation and commitment to help fellow human beings using a particular expertise based on a body of esoteric knowledge, who would always put the interests of the clients first and not seek to exploit their vulnerability. But are these traditional values still held today, have they changed and, if so, can we throw any light on why or how this might have happened?

My starting point is the proposition that doctors' behaviour is just as much a function of the structure of the situation in which they practise as it is a consequence of how they have been trained or socialized. Of interest for our purpose here is the possibility that changes in the status and power of doctors, real or perceived, will be reflected in the way that values are espoused and enacted in practice. A second proposition to be considered is that there is a dynamic relationship between values and practice (expressed either in words or actions), and that it can run in either direction. By that I mean that values may exert a powerful influence on behaviour but, equally, there may be a strong push for individuals to accommodate and adjust their values to fit what they find themselves actually doing in a particular situation (Pattison and Pill 2004).

Following a brief account of the development of British general practice, these propositions are explored by focusing on the interaction between the way in which UK health care is organized and the day-to-day context in which GPs work, and how this affects the way they perceive their role, present themselves to others, and their actual practice.

GPS AND THE NATIONAL HEALTH SERVICE 1948–74

When the National Health Service was introduced in 1948 the medical profession was greatly opposed to local government control of the health service since this smacked too much of the control over doctors exercised by working men in the 'sick clubs' that had provided much of the health care up till then (see Stacey 1988). The consensus was that the hospital doctors overall did rather better out of the negotiations than GPs as they were given guaranteed salaries and financial incentives while retaining the right to do private practice. The GPs had no intention of becoming the salaried servants of anyone and argued to remain as independent entrepreneurs, paid according to a capitation system based on the old National Insurance Scheme and controlled by a local committee of doctors with limited lay membership. The GPs usually worked alone, often from home, with minimal administrative support. These arrangements perpetuated the division between hospital doctors and GPs and altered their relationship, since the former were no longer so financially dependent on the latter referring private patients to them. In the years following GPs have been described as being:

> an isolated and defensive group who had lost interest in challenging the dominance of the hospital specialists. Their professional development was at a standstill and in many respects their poor conditions of work, low income and long hours of work were the price they were paying for owning

> their own practice and being independent. Their position can
> be likened to the small shopkeeper. (Calnan and Gabe 1991,
> p.144)

Pressure for improved conditions of service culminated in the threat of mass resignations in the 1960s and finally resulted in a new 'GP charter' in 1965. This heralded not only a change in working conditions but also significant changes in the organization of general practice, e.g. new health centres, a trend towards larger practices, more extensive use of appointment systems and a new concept of the primary health care team (Wilkin *et al.* 1987).

A debate emerged about content and quality of general practitioner care between those advocating a more traditional clinical approach, modelled closely on hospital medical practice, and those in favour of a more social orientation and the development of a distinct and new body of knowledge (Calnan 1988). The former position was advocated by the General Medical Services Committee of the British Medical Association (the body that acts as the doctors' trade union), which argued that GPs should be given the resources to develop their skills and extend their range of activities into areas such as minor surgery. In contrast to this a more holistic approach was advocated (and supported by the leaders of the now *Royal* College of General Practitioners) in which the focus was on understanding signs and symptoms in the context of the patient's own biography and environment and extending the GPs' role into health promotion and disease (Balint and Norell 1973; Calnan and Gabe 1991; Hart 1984).

The reforms of 1974 unified the three arms of the NHS, namely, public health, hospital services and general practice, and introduced the concept of responsibility upwards to managerial authority. As noted in Chapter 1, however, doctors succeeded in retaining 'clinical autonomy' so that they could be fully responsible for the treatment they prescribed for patients. Thus, unlike all other health workers, they were exempted from direct managerial control. Moreover, GPs who had improved their pay, status and working conditions in 1965 insisted on retaining essentially the same structure that they had originally brought into the NHS, now to be called Family Practitioner Committees.

THE TRANSFORMATION OF PRIMARY CARE: 1974 TO THE PRESENT DAY

The introduction of the internal market and GP fundholding initiative (GPFH) under the Conservative government in the 1980s and 1990s (see Chapter 1) has been described as an attempt to introduce consumer choice and competition into health care by balancing what was perceived to be a previously unequal relationship between GPs and hospital doctors in determining the operation of the health service. Although the evidence is mixed on the benefits and, more particularly, on the cost effectiveness achieved by GPFH (Coulter 1995) the improved integration and continuity of care and the increased leverage over hospital services acquired by GPs through their new commissioning powers (Glennester, Matasaganis and Owens 1994; Klein 1995) was recognized by the New Labour administration that gained power in 1997.[1]

The drive for primary care to assume a much greater coordinating function in the health service has now been central to health reform for nearly two decades (Frusher 2006). In the White Paper (Department of Health 1997) the purchaser–provider split was retained and a mechanism established to retain GPs' involvement in the commissioning process by creating primary care groups (PCGs) in 1999. The hope was that these groups would maintain the service improvements pioneered by fundholding. By 2002 these were re-invented as primary care trusts (PCTs) and tasked with combining both purchasing and provision functions, thus assuming responsibility for commissioning care that spanned the health, social care and independent sectors. Primary care clinicians were given a majority standing on professional executive committees of PCTs, thus providing them with a much greater formal role in setting strategy and directing the organization. Practice-based commissioning was introduced in order to encourage devolved decision-making. The importance attached to primary care was further demonstrated by the decision to allot PCTs a unified budget that equated to 75–80% of the entire health care budget. Such a transformation necessarily has, and will continue to have, a considerable impact on GPs, whose function now

---

1   For reasons of space and clarity this chapter focuses specifically on the developments in health services in England since the establishment of the NHS and the reactions of GPs in that part of the UK to the changes over this period, and speculates on the implications for this group of professionals. It is recognized, of course, that the other smaller countries that comprise the UK have adopted different approaches, particularly since devolution, and the pattern of change (and hence the context in which GPs are working) shows increasing variation, offering fascinating potential for comparison (see Greer and Rowland 2007).

has been defined as prime coordinators of care and as managers of the local health economy (Frusher 2006).

There can be no doubt that, since the mid-1980s, the State has become very interested in general practice for economic, political and ideological reasons. One reason already considered is the wish to restrict/achieve better control over public spending. Other commentators have pointed out the desire to make individual consumer choice the dominant value in welfare policy, and perhaps also to curtail the power of the professions (Calnan and Gabe 1991). GP reaction to these developments can be traced in the professional journals, especially the editorials and letter pages over the past 20 years, which chronicle an increasingly heated debate about the implications of the changes being implemented or proposed for professionals and their clients. It is hardly surprising that there is a wide spectrum of opinion given the differences already noted in the two schools of thought about the way that the GP role should evolve; the tensions between hospital doctors and general practitioners and, within general practice itself; and the potential for disagreement between the élite, academics and medical politicians often largely based in London, and the rest of the working GPs.

VALUES DISCOURSE

Here our interest is in the extent to which GPs themselves explored or discussed values or recognized that their values might be changing or under attack in a changing environment. The focus is on the discourse of values, the definition of values (Howie, Heaney and Maxwell 2004; Irvine 2004; Pringle 1998) and the circumstances in which they are invoked. Examination of the discourse in 'official documents', i.e. the statements and responses to government policy documents made by professional bodies, is particularly useful for this purpose. Inspection can reveal not only which values are claimed explicitly but also the implicit values underpinning arguments and, perhaps even more important, the ways in which each document seeks to persuade a larger audience of the validity of these arguments. So, when considering where 'values talk' might be found we can distinguish the internal debates within each group (to be found in professional journals and publications) from the more formal statements issued by the Royal Colleges and other professional bodies in response to government policy initiatives and directives. After all, such documents are produced in the knowledge that they will be scrutinized by other health professionals, administrators, media and academic commentators and the public in general. They form part of an ongoing process within the UK health sector as each occupational group seeks to maintain, extend and assert their position relative to others, while, at the same time, they are attempting to reject, modify or accept the changes proposed and being implemented by central government and the local health trusts. Therefore it is likely that there will be differences in emphasis, refutations and counter-claims as time goes by and the context changes, particularly in a situation where administrations have been determined to push forward with radical reform of the NHS over the past two decades.

The Royal College of General Practitioners

The Royal College of General Practitioners (RCGP), founded only in 1952, is a relatively young organization compared with the Royal Colleges of other medical specialities. Milestones in its history include the establishment of vocational training in general practice, the setting up of clinical guidelines for doctors, the expansion of research into general medical practice and the promotion of multi-disciplinary primary care. Today, the RCGP is a network of around 26,000 doctors (representing over half of all UK GPs, based on data collated by the RCGP in 2006) who are committed to improving patient care, developing their own skills and developing general practice (RCGP2006). Membership, which is not mandatory, is open to doctors who have passed one of a number of specified assesments, and illustrations of the content and style of some recent statements are given below.

In 2001 the College, together with the GP committee of the British Medical Association (BMA) and the NHS Alliance, produced a paper titled *Valuing General Practice* in response to proposals in the NHS Plan for England that were felt to impact on the core values of general practice, its quality and training, and hence on its ability to deliver high-quality patient care. The following key statements were set out in response to the perceived challenges posed by the NHS plan and appropriate justifications provided. For example:

- Primary care is an essential feature of an efficient and effective health care system.

- General practice and general practitioners have a unique and important contribution to make to primary care and the NHS. Flexibility in professional boundaries may change some working practices, but the vital central role of the GP cannot be substituted by others.

- Increased investment in primary care, including general practice, will yield better patient outcomes with more efficient use of resources.

- The variation in quality within primary care is unacceptable. Major efforts must be made to improve the experience of all patients so that unacceptable practice is eliminated.

(RCGP 2001, p.3)

The amplification of the second point is particularly relevant in setting out their concept of the role of the GP in relation to other primary care professionals. For example, 'enhanced nurse roles, including nurse prescribing' are supported and a proposal for the development of the community pharmacist within primary care teams mentioned. However, while it is stated that flexibility of roles *must* take into account core competencies, the most appropriate carer and efficiency, doubts are also expressed about the opportunity costs of extended roles for nurses in the erosion of traditional nursing skills that are highly valued by patients and by nurses' professional colleagues.

The unique and key attributes of the GP that should be valued are listed as follows:

- *Complex clinical skills and high-level communication skills.* The capacity to deploy these skills in a short, ten minute consultation requires a breadth of biomedical and psychosocial knowledge and the complexity of the role, the gate keeper between perceived illness and disease, must not be underestimated.

- *Flexibility.* GPs reformulate their care to meet the needs of individual patients as they evolve, offering personally tailored care including the right access to the right parts of the health service when appropriate.

- *Continuity of care.* Seeing a doctor who knows the patient and remembers key events in the life of that patient and the family, who will be there subsequently when required and who takes a longer term view of care and its outcomes is an important feature of primary care work.

(RCGP 2001, pp.6–7)

In September 2004 a second paper, *The Future of General Practice*, was produced by the then chairman of the College council and 'a small group of thoughtful and influential GPs' (RCGP 2004). In the Introduction the chairman said that he felt it essential to be able to 'state clearly and concisely what our value and our values are', and that he wanted the document to be read, to trigger discussion and debate. The background is described as follows:

It has been a worrying time for many general practitioners. Do we have a future or are we an unwanted anachronism? Over the past few years medical newspapers have regularly carried stories about threats to our role in the NHS. Many individual doctors have expressed genuine concern that their job is changing beyond recognition, that there is a covert agenda to replace GPs with other care professionals and that our days are numbered. (RCGP 2004, p.2)

This document builds on the unique skills of GPs set out in *Valuing General Practice* and emphasizes that public confidence in GPs is remarkably high, notwithstanding a small number of highly publicized scandals, and that, as generalist physicians, GPs are even more relevant in dealing with increasing numbers of older patients with co-morbidities. Again, it is argued that coordination of care, the personalizing of care to individual need and the delivery of the majority of that care must reside with a physician who knows and understands the individual patient, and the conclusion is drawn that it is essential that the medical generalist of the future offers high-quality medical care without losing the attributes of being patient-centred, listening, caring and trusted.

The authors of the RCGP document accept the need for flexible, patient-centred models of care delivery, including more rapid access to medical care, and also recognize that technological advances, near-patient diagnostics (in which tests are carried out as near to the patient as possible, including in the home) and minimally invasive interventions will have a major impact on delivery. Yet they stress that new models of access must not damage the possibility of a patient choosing continuity of care with an individual GP if that is that patient's priority. Their conclusion is that organizational change should support the development of practices and the medical generalist since the more complicated the world becomes, the more the GP will be needed. Thus the current situation of overcrowding in outpatient departments and inappropriate use of secondary care can be minimized and overall care for the nation's patients will be improved, highly accessible and personalized (RCGP 2004, pp.4–7).

The above examples display the views of the professional body of GPs on their particular expertise and why it should be valued by policymakers and those responsible for organizing health services. Like other professional groups they lay claim to a particular aspect of patient care but, in contrast to ever narrower specialization, they stress the value of a holistic long-term relationship based on trust. As for relations to the other primary care professionals the emphasis is on teamwork, with the claim being made for the GP to have a key coordinating role. What is striking is that there is no mention of concepts found in the earlier literature on the professions such as 'exclusive bodies of knowledge' or 'autonomy', which were felt to define the ideal type of a professional. Instead, there are specific references to the changes in the context of care and emphasis on new forms of practice reflecting different values. Thus instead of the model of the often single-handed, rather isolated GP who has a paternalistic, or even authoritarian, attitude towards his patients we are presented with a team leader who is readier to negotiate with clients about their needs and treatment.

I suggest that what these papers illustrate is that the RCGP is attempting a delicate balancing act. It is not only trying to stake and maintain its position in relation to other professional groups in the health field but also to negotiate with the shifts in policy and demands made by the politicians and bureaucrats. What is being implicitly valued in these recent responses are not the old values of professionalization theory but those coming from the field of organization theory, namely: the capacity to work effectively as a member of a team, to relate to clients as partners in the health project, or even as consumers with the right to choose; the need to justify practice in terms of outcomes; to provide value for money and improved effectiveness and efficiency. These reflect, in turn, the changing government policies put forward in recent White Papers:

> This White Paper sets a new direction for the whole health and social care system. It confirms the vision set out in the Department of Health Green Paper, *Independence, Wellbeing and Choice*. There will be a radical and sustained shift in the way in which services are delivered, ensuring that they are more personalised and that they fit into people's busy lives. We will give people a stronger voice so that they are the major drivers of service improvement. (Department of Health 2006, p.1)

On the one hand, the RCGP has appealed to the past, stressing what a good job GPs have been doing, and how important general practice is to the delivery of quality primary care where the bulk of NHS work is done. On the other, it is presenting itself as ready to cooperate and adapt where necessary. A parallel underlying theme has been that we are not appreciated (valued?) enough, and this cry has become shriller in the past couple of years (Haslam 2003) as recruitment became more difficult not only in the UK (Evans, Lambert and Goldacre 2002) but also in other English-speaking countries (Del Mar, Freeman and van Weel 2003; Rosser 2002).

However, in one of the latest statements by the RCGP (2007) there has been an interesting change of tone. Here, instead of reacting to an official policy, the College (in association with a wide range of other GP bodies and other medical colleges) puts forward its own ideas for the development of general practice and patient care in a document designed to be used to 'influence, support and challenge policymakers at national and local levels'. The claim is made that a new model of health and social care is required that builds on the needs of patients and the strengths and values of general practice. The executive summary reiterates concisely the case for general practice but goes on to outline the potential for collaborative groupings of practices and specifically rejects the notion of the 'polyclinic', as proposed by Lord Darzi in his review of the London Services:

> The practice and the primary health care team must remain the basic unit of care. This federated model of general practice, championed and led by GPs, is essential to counter the challenges of a 'market' approach in the NHS, a particular concern in England. (RCGP 2007, executive summary, p.2)

One reaction to statements such as the ones above might be 'Well, they would say that, wouldn't they!' Of course, the question arises as to whether these documents are simply political rhetoric reflecting the self-interests of a London-based élite and to what extent they can be said to reflect the views of the whole body of GPs. There is an obvious difference between the activities of a corporate body claiming to represent the profession and the activities of an aggregate of individual general practitioners. Nevertheless, professional organizations perform a useful function in providing the professions with a distinct ideology that can be used at the official level, even if it may not be accepted by a large segment of working GPs (Calnan and Gabe 1991).

THE FUTURE: TRENDS AND IMPLICATIONS
New contracts and a changing workforce
In the past 20 years there have been considerable changes to the organization and content of GPs' work. For example, the increasing use of deputizing services had begun to erode the concept of cradle-to-grave, 24-hour care from a particular doctor before the Department of Health in 1990 (being unable to reach agreement with a reluctant profession) imposed a contract that substantially reduced clinical freedom. Practices were required to produce annual reports, three-yearly health checks for adults and annual checks for older patients, while prescribing was constrained through the introduction of limited lists and indicative drug budgets. It has been argued that subsequent negotiations resulting in the new 2004 contract represent the trade-offs between those aspects that were perceived by the GPs as reducing workload (such as shedding out of hours responsibilities) and enhancing salaries and those that constrained clinical freedom, such as targets and bureaucracy (see Iliffe 2008). Now it is the NHS, not the GP, that offers the service and the local Primary Care Trust that 'owns' the patients and their records.

Before thinking about the impact of these processes on values and practice we need also to be aware of the changes in the characteristics of the workforce. In 1983, 98% of GPs in England worked as full-time principals; by 2004, 41% of GPs were classified as non-principals (non-principals are either locums, retainers (most often women with family commitments) or salaried GPs (referred to as associates prior to 2004)) and over one-fifth of the principals were part-time (Department of Health 2004). Some clues to the dramatic increase of non-principals may be found in a longitudinal study of the careers of 544 doctors graduating in 1995 (Jones and Fisher 2006). It was found that while general practice was not initially attractive to this sample it became popular later as offering a superior work–life balance and that, once in general practice, both male and female doctors chose to work reduced hours and/or in non-principal posts.

Since 1948 GPs had always been 'independent contractors' to the State, rather than employees. But nobody has thought of them as being in the private sector, and they enjoyed a generous NHS pension. Recently, four new contracting options were introduced, each of which is between the government or local health commissioners and health care companies. The fourth option, one that marks off this reform from earlier revisions, allows commercial companies to hold the provider contract. GPs will be under contract to companies or trusts and not the State.

Commentators have pointed out that this introduces the concept of privatization into primary care (Pollock 2006; Smith 2005). Services are being broken up into saleable commodities; clinical decision-making shared with the primary care team will come under the control of commercial managers and shareholders (some of whom will be GP shareholders) (Pollock 2006). It seems likely that there will be considerable division of opinion among GPs about the opportunities and implications of these latest developments, some welcoming the commercial possibilities and the ending of an 'open-ended commitment to care' with its inevitable constraints on time and energy, while others are less sure (Iliffe 2008). What is clear is that GPs will have a greater variety of work settings to choose from and will presumably seek an environment that they feel fits best with their own personal and professional values and the way they want to practise. There is already some intriguing evidence about possible developments in this direction.

The 'new general practice'?

Jones and Green (2006) interviewed 20 early-career GPs who had graduated in 1995, the majority of whom were working as non-principals, i.e. receiving a salary and not as partners in a practice (they were selected from the BMA cohort study mentioned above). In a labour market then characterized by problems in GP recruitment and policy initiatives to attract more GPs, the GPs in this study had secured favourable contracts and, perhaps unsurprisingly, reported extremely high job satisfaction. This contrasted with much earlier work in primary care in the past 20 years that was characterized by reports of poor morale. These GPs had found 'nice work': preferably undertaken in friendly, well-run, innovative practices that allowed them considerable control over hours of work; the combination of GP work and either non-work interests or other professional interests; and the kind of general practice undertaken (Jones and Green 2006).

However, most were careful to present themselves as not seeking to avoid the well-known stress of general practice through 'dropping out' or making purely self-serving decisions to prioritize their own quality of life. Instead, their decisions were presented as constituting a 'new' professionalism, entailing the rejection of some core values of traditional professionalism and the re-framing of others. Most striking was the de-coupling of a sense of vocation from professionalism:

> We found a carefulness on the part of these GPs to present their work as 'professional' in that it was practised in a way which maximised benefits to patients. Indeed, given the changing health care environment their orientations to work were presented as <u>better</u> able to meet the needs of patients than 'traditional' models of practice... Vocation was explicitly associated with 'old-fashioned attitudes', which were framed not only as anachronistic, but also potentially damaging in both the paternalism they engendered in relationships with clients and the unhealthy self sacrifice demanded by continuous access to patients. Old-fashioned vocation extended a dominance over other areas of life that was inherently problematic, rather than morally wanting. (Jones and Green 2006, p.944)

What is clear here is that these GPs still see themselves as 'professionals', albeit bearing different meanings and responsibilities from previous notions of professional practice (Lupton 1997). Like other professionals, doctors are less likely now to work as solo practitioners or in partnerships that last for a working life and are more likely to find themselves in complex or novel organizations. The different orientation of this group of early career GPs, compared with that of the traditional, full-time principal rooted in a community, provide an interesting example of the way in which individuals can construct/reconstruct their notions of professional identity.

The new GP-manager?

Another possible path for the GP, one that we have seen to be strongly encouraged by the government in the transformed, ever-changing primary care system, is involvement in the management of the local health economy. One view has been that professionals *are* taking on more managerial roles, thereby retaining their professional ethos but doing so to the backdrop of the managerial discourse engendered by the new status conferred on primary care (Causer and Exworthy 1999). Other commentators have queried the extent to which GPs will be able to develop an effective balance between the managerial needs of the health system and their everyday clinical practice. While effective primary care is promoted as the key driver to delivering coordinated, integrated care, GPs who are customarily best placed to oversee this are experiencing changes to the system that might prevent them from doing so successfully. For example, the traditional 'gatekeeping' function is now being eroded with the diversification of primary care, as there is now an increasingly varied number of ways for patients to access health professionals, e.g. NHS Direct, walk-in centres. Thus, while GPs are provided with a range of tools and mechanisms to commission more integrated pathways, their own position in the continuum of care is potentially undermined.

The responsibility for maintaining care pathways will be exercised most strongly through GPs' commissioning role, at an individual practice level and as part of the wider health economy. Such responsibility has as its root a clinical focus, with clinicians ensuring that the patient's navigation through the health system determines the best clinical outcome. However, 'as these networks develop across primary care there is a concomitant increase in financial complexity and GPs, as practice-based commissioners, will be required to understand the financial flows that constitute their local health economies' (Frusher 2006, p.52).

The position will be further complicated by the underlying pressure to contain costs. This will inevitably heighten GPs' potential conflict of interest between serving the best interests of individual patients and serving the wider public need by containing costs. Frusher (2006) points out that, although rationing has often been implicit and unquestioned, increasing challenges to specific treatment decisions are likely to raise public awareness of the resource-allocation role and put GPs and their practices, as managers of the local health economy and the underlying rationing process, under much greater scrutiny.

The question arises as to whether there is the organizational capacity available to meet all these new necessary management functions as well as meeting the demands of policy and expectations of patients. In order to be effective commissioners, practices will be required to monitor performance of existing services and acquire and manage the information needed to develop new ones. Practices will also need to work with PCTs in order to manage instances of service failure and poor delivery of care so as to ensure continuity and quality of provision. But, as Frusher points out, 'it is not clear that the appropriate level of management resources and required volume of expertise necessary for these decision to be made reliably is currently widely accessible anywhere in primary care' (Frusher 2006, p.54). The recent report published by the King's Fund supports these reservations, warning that the government must commit to a fundamental reassessment of the policy and tackle the waning enthusiasm among GPs if it is to build on the limited progress the scheme has made (Curry *et al.* 2008). It remains to be seen to what extent GPs will be prepared to adapt to a new role as a managerial-professional.

Changes in the nature of general practice work

Parallel with organizational changes described earlier there have also been profound changes in the nature of medical work carried out by GPs and practice nurses over the past 20 years. For example, in 1990 the then Conservative government imposed a new contract on generally reluctant GPs requiring them to undertake screening measures on groups of patients in order to earn a proportion of their income. As Checkland (2004) comments:

> whilst 20 years ago the majority of activity within a practice consisted of patient-initiated contacts in response to their own perception of their need, most modern General Practices, as well as providing appointments for those who ask for them, provide a parallel service of ongoing and preventative care to patients according to a programme. (p.953)

The demands associated with providing these two kinds of service are very different and the need for acute care has not lessened as the provision of chronic-disease management has increased. The introduction of National Service Frameworks (NSFs) in 1997 went beyond simply providing guidelines about appropriate clinical care for individual patients to supply detailed preferred 'service models' that laid down how, and by whom, that care should be delivered. It is now an explicit duty of the Primary Care Trusts to report on the extent to which NSFs are being implemented and there is a clear presumption from central government that this will become the norm. The 2004 contract for GPs institutionalizes these changes further 'with a significant proportion of GP income being dependent upon the attainment of a large number of detailed quality indicators that embody the concept of organised care of those with chronic disease according to normative guidelines' (Checkland 2004, p.954).

This 'scientific-bureaucratic' approach (Harrison 2002) is more closely identified with public health and a clinic-based approach to groups of patients than with traditional general practice and its emphasis on holistic care of the individual. So, how are GPs on the ground coping with these changes in their everyday work situation and the demands being made on them? Here again an ethnographic approach using qualitative methods can throw light on what is actually happening in the daily decision-making and the practical mechanisms by which medicine is delivered to patients.

Drawing on the work of Lipsky (1980) and his concept of public service workers as 'street-level bureaucrats', Checkland (2004, p.954) argues that as 'well as being professionals doctors are also workers who, like other workers, are active agents, negotiating the terms of their daily existence in unique ways across a variety of work situations.' This approach focuses on how GPs make sense of their daily work while constructing understandings that normalize their lives as workers and allow them to cope with uncertainty. It is argued that GPs are like many public service workers who interact directly with people in the course of their jobs and share the following characteristics:

- a need to process workloads expeditiously;

- substantial autonomy in their individual interactions with clients;

- an interest in maintaining and maximizing that autonomy;
- conditions of work that include inadequate resources (both monetary, and in terms of personnel and time);
- demand that will always exceed supply;
- ambiguous and multiple objectives;
- difficulties in defining or measuring good performance;
- a need to take rapid decisions for clients who have a limited or non-existent choice over whether, where or how they present to the service involved.

(Checkland 2004, pp.955–957)

Lipsky proposed that the decisions public-service workers make in response to such pressures, the routines they establish, and the devices they invent to cope with uncertainties and work pressures become the public policies they carry out. This process has been identified in a study of GP decision-making about the management of coronary heart disease patients where the practical decisions were at odds with stated local policy (McDonald 2002). Similarly, there are Checkland's own case studies of general practices that, although having a track record of adopting clinical guidelines, nevertheless did not take on board National Service Frameworks. She comments that 'more studies at this micro-level focusing on the sense that individuals make of their working lives may contribute to deeper understanding of the complex responses to centrally-imposed change' (p.972).

At the start of this chapter it was argued that we need to recognize that values are just as likely to be the product of changing organization and circumstances as to be the driving force for practice (see also Klein 2007). The increasing importance placed in primary care by successive governments, coupled with the growth of regulation and the 'audit culture', has dramatically altered the work conditions and resources available to GPs in the past 20 years. As medicine became more and more specialized and fragmented, particularly in the hospital sector, there are signs that GPs are also beginning to query and redefine their traditional roles as 'gatekeepers to secondary care' and 'generalists'. In response to increasing state interventions and the rapid rate of change in the wider NHS system, GPs appear to have collectively responded by shifting their 'values' to ensure some preservation of existing occupational advantages as well as traditions of work.

As for the future, what cannot be doubted is that doctors completing the mandatory training to become GPs today have a much wider range of possible work settings to choose from (including going abroad) and will seek to construct their identity amid a variety of options in a rapidly changing health care system. Their choice of setting may reflect their values at the time and their experiences in any given setting may also influence the values they come to hold and their behaviour.

RESPONSE
Paquita de Zulueta

The author of this chapter makes two key propositions: first, that professional behaviours relate just as much to the context in which individuals work as to their training and socialization; second, that values and practice are in a dynamic relationship to one another, such that individuals accommodate their values to 'fit' their actual behaviours (and vice versa). These propositions carry with them the important implication that the professed values of general practice could be profoundly affected by the current socio-political climate, and that GPs' actual day-to-day working practices more accurately reflect *their* values, rather than those expressed in official documents.

We are provided with a concise and useful summary of the development of general practice as a speciality in its own right, complete with its own core values and training requirements. The claim, however, that the reforms of the 1980s and 1990s resulted in 'improved integration and continuity of care' is highly questionable. I believe that the various changes, as described above, in fact combined to *reduce* continuity of care. Furthermore, the increased leverage over hospital services was partial and limited to fundholding general practices. I would also adopt a more critical stance towards the term 'purchaser–provider split' in the context of primary care, as GPs can act as both purchasers and providers. Indeed, setting financial rewards for providing services 'in-house' can create conflicts of interest that remain undisclosed or unacknowledged. The increased responsibility for cost containment also creates an ethical conflict between serving the best interests of individual patients versus those of the wider community – a conflict that GPs may not be so familiar with or recognizant of (Smith and Morrisey 1994).

The author suggests that the values expressed in the documents *Valuing General practice* (RCGP 2001) and *The Future of General practice* (RCGP 2004) may represent the views of an élite (consisting of academics and medical politicians) rather than those of working GPs. But since the education of GPs closely reflects these values, I think that this allegation is at best only partially true. These documents give us, she says, a new concept of professionalism, with greater emphasis on doctor–patient partnership and clinical outcomes and with a reduced paternalism. This represents, in her view, an attempt by the profession (championed by the Royal College of General Practitioners or RCGP) 'not only... to stake and maintain its position in relation to other professional groups...but also to negotiate with the shifts in policy and demands made by the politicians and bureaucrats'. I would venture an alternative interpretation: that the authors of these documents are endeavouring to stick to their guns (values!) because they perceive threats to these longstanding, and presumably deeply cherished, values – some of which have been articulated for at least 40 years. The key attributes cited in these documents – the capacity to deliver individualized, patient-centred holistic care, an emphasis on continuity and coordination of care, and the enactment of complex clinical skills and high levels of communication skills – are not new. In fact, if one looks at the much earlier document, *The Future General Practitioner* (RCGP 1972), one finds – albeit expressed differently – virtually the same values and attributes.

The key changes in the delivery of general practice starting since the reforms in 1990 are instrumental in creating this divergence. I will briefly comment on a few described by the author in the delivery of general practice since the reforms of 1990. The description by Jones and Green (2006) of a large cohort of contented, part-time, salaried GPs working within a 'sellers' market' – assertive professionals able to dictate the terms and conditions of their work – does not fit with the current realities. We now have an excess of trained general practitioners competing for jobs in the market, a deepening of the partner/non-partner divide, and anecdotal evidence of exploitation of a 'flexible workforce'. This insecure workforce is more likely to be compliant and less assertive. It is a moot point whether GPs will have the luxury to practise in an environment that is compatible with their personal and professional values, particularly as some of their employers will be large private organizations that may well not share these.

I would also question the view that vocation has been uncoupled from professionalism. If 'vocation' is defined as limitless boundaries, neglect of personal needs and the welfare of one's immediate family, then I can agree. But vocation is more than that – it can be viewed as a calling to use one's talents and skills in the service of others. It does not need to be total self-sacrifice. Griffin (2008) gives an alternative view of professionalism and describes a reprofessionalization rather than a deprofessionalization process, with the integration of multiple conceptual frameworks and roles in her work as a 'portfolio doctor'.

I would also like to comment on the impact of performance-related pay in the shape of the Quality and Outcomes Framework (QOF). Mangin and Toop (2007, p.436), describe QOF as a 'disempowering system of micro-management' that corrodes ethical practice and professionalism. Undoubtedly, QOF carries the risks of 'tick-box medicine', of a top-down agenda that eclipses that of the patient's, and the intrinsic professional motivation to benefit patients being undermined by externally imposed incentives (McDonald *et al.* 2007). But Lester and Roland (2007) take the view that the use of incentives to improve quality of care has been beneficial. They do acknowledge, however, that prizing the easily measurable and financially rewarding ('QOFable') activities carries the risk of deprioritizing the less measurable and definable aspects of care – and arguably this will include much of the 'hidden work' of general practice. The pernicious effect of putting a price tag on every clinical activity and allowing money to be the driver of change has also been commented on by Iona Heath who bemoans the loss of altruism in public service (Heath 2007).

In summary, the changes in general practice can be viewed as a transition from relative autonomy to a much closer linkage with the health care state. The active management of general practice, gathering momentum from the 1990s onwards, reflects government policy to control primary care such that it 'delivers' a high-quality, more homogeneous service that is accessible, flexible and efficient. This has been accompanied by a drive to increase transparency, accountability and access as well as a broadening of the scope of general practice to include more chronic-disease management, disease prevention and health promotion. These changes can also be viewed as a shift from a public service model to an industrialized market-based model of health care (Iliffe 2008; Tudor-

Hart 2006) or the adoption of Harrison's 'scientific-bureaucratic model' (Harrison 2002).

Values have been described as 'normal', that is to say assumed and central to personal and social identity, or 'aspirational', that is to say consciously sought after (Pattison 2004). If we take the RCGP model to be aspirational, the key question is how close is it to the model that is actually enacted 'on the ground'? And, if there *is* a divergence (and I argue that there is), how wide is that gap? We also need to ask how sustainable are these aspirational values, if we find that professional behaviours are regularly in conflict with them? In order to answer these questions we rely on ethnographic research and anecdotal evidence.

Charles-Jones, Latimer and May (2003), in their illuminating qualitative study, address the question of how GPs have responded to the extra workload and responsibility placed upon them whilst managing patient demand. The authors propose that primary care practice emerges as increasingly concerned with managerial systems of efficiency rather than people: 'Crucially, the effect is to move the focus of general practice work to biomedical aspects of a patient's problem and redistribute responsibility for the patient's narrative to those with the least expertise' (Charles-Jones *et al.* 2003, p.82). GPs are found to maintain their high professional status by reconfiguring themselves as 'specialists' or consultants and sustain hierarchical differences by segregating and extending the nurses' roles. Patients are categorized according to a set of criteria dictated by the practice. The social and psychological aspects of their condition are marginalized, with the exception of those with mental health problems or terminally ill. 'The patient becomes less of a person and more of a biomedical diagnosis to be managed in the system' (Charles-Jones *et al.* 2003, p.84). The GP moves out of the fuzzy space of 'old' general practice into a more 'purist biomedical space' that is more sharply delineated, more readily circumscribed and managed. The GP, in turn, 'is located in (and by) the technologies of efficiency and transparency – the computer and the audit' (Charles-Jones *et al.* 2003, p.85).

In conclusion, my understanding is that there is a widening gulf between the normal and aspirational models of general practice. The manner in which GPs are behaving in the workplace does not reflect the values that they are said to espouse: patient-centred care, sustained partnership in the doctor–patient relationship, and whole-person medicine. To this we could add empathy (Howie *et al.* 2004). What we appear to have instead is a heavy emphasis on public health priorities, the rhetoric of 'choice', persistence of short appointment times, an increased fragmentation and discontinuity of care, and a more compartmentalized, disease-focused, and impersonal model of care. Despite this rather bleak conclusion, one can remind oneself that GPs have shown their resilience and independent thinking in the past. Let us hope that they are still capable of it now. Patients themselves may successfully champion a more holistic, patient-centred approach. Another glimmer of hope lies, paradoxically, in the collapse of the financial market and its accompanying global recession. Given that the promulgation of human vices such as greed and selfishness has been the hallmark of the poorly regulated market, perhaps people will begin to acknowledge that systems fostering the 'old-fashioned' human virtues might be more fitting for an intrinsically moral enterprise such as medicine? The hand of solidarity, support and succour extended to those in need may represent a more fitting symbol than the very invisible hand of the market.

REFERENCES

Balint, E. and Norell, J.S. (1973) *Six Minutes for the Patient: Interactions in the General Consultation.* London: Tavistock.

Calnan, M. (1988) 'Variations in the range of services provided by GPs.' *Family Practice 5,* 2, 904–104.

Calnan, M. and Gabe, J. (1991) 'Recent developments in General practice.' In M. Calnan, J. Gabe and M. Bury (eds) *The Sociology of the Health Service.* London: Routledge.

Causer, G. and Exworthy, M. (1999) 'Professionals as Managers across the Public Sector.' In M. Exworthy and S. Halford (eds) *Professionals and the New Managerialism in the Public Sector.* Buckingham: Open University Press.

Charles-Jones, H., Latimer, J. and May, C. (2003) 'Transforming General practice: the redistribution of medical work in primary care.' *Sociology of Health and Illness 25,* 1, 71–92.

Checkland, K. (2004) 'National Service Frameworks and UK general practitioners: street-level bureaucrats at work?' *Sociology of Health and Illness 20,* 7, 951–975.

Curry, N., Goodwin, N., Naylor, C. and Robertson, R. (2008) *Practice-based Commissioning: Reinvigorate, Replace or Abandon?* London: The King's Fund.

Coulter, A. (1995) 'Evaluating General practice fund-holding in the UK.' *European Journal of Public Health 5,* 3, 233–239.

Del Mar, C.B., Freeman, G.K. and van Weel, C. (2003) '"Only a GP?": is the solution to the General practice crisis intellectual?' *Medical Journal of Australia 179,* 1, 26–29.

Department of Health (1997) *The New NHS: Modern, Dependable.* London: The Stationery Office.

Department of Health (2004) *Statistics for General Medical Practitioners for England 1993–2003. Bulletin 2004/3.* London: Department of Health.

Department of Health (2006) *Our Health, Our Care, Our Say: a New Direction for Community Services.* London: Department of Health.

Evans, J., Lambert, T. and Goldacre, M. (2002) 'GP Recruitment and Retention: A Qualitative Analysis of Doctors' Comments about Training for and Working in General practice.' *Occasional Paper 83.* London: RCGP.

Frusher, T. (2006) 'Managing change: General practice and the transformation of primary care.' *Health Policy Review, 3,* 44–58.

Glennester, H., Matasaganis, M. and Owens, S. (1994) *Implementing GP Fundholding.* Buckingham: Open University Press.

Greer, L.S. and Rowland, D. (2007) *Devolving Policy, Diverging Values: The Values of the United Kingdom's National Health Services.* London: The Nuffield Trust

Griffin, A. (2008) 'Designer doctors: professional identity and a portfolio career as a General practice educator.' *Education for Primary Care 19,* 4, 355–359.

Harrison, S. (2002) 'New Labour, modernization and the medical labour process.' *Journal of Social Policy 31,* 3, 465–485.

Hart, J.T. (1984) 'Still nobody's business? Prevention of coronary disease through primary care.' *Practitioner 228,* 41–50.

Haslam, D. (2003) 'GPs on the critical list. Why are the family doctors so undervalued when they are so crucial to the health of the nation?' *The Observer,* Sunday 13 April 2003. Available at www.guardian.co.uk/society/2003/apr/13/medicineandhealth.comment, accessed on 12 March 2009.

Heath, I. (2007) 'Something rotten.' *British Medical Journal 335,* 7625, 855.

Howie, J.G.R., Heaney, D. and Maxwell, M. (2004) 'Quality, core values and General practice consultation: issues of definition, measurement and delivery.' *Family Practice 21,* August, 458–468.

Iliffe, S. (2008) *From General practice to Primary Care: the Industrialisation of Family Medicine.* Oxford: Oxford University Press.

Irvine, D. (2004) '17th Gordon Arthur Ransome Oration: patient-centred professionalism.' *Annals Academy of Medicine 33,* 6, 680–685.

Jones, L. and Green, J. (2006) 'Shifting discourses of professionalism: a case study of general practitioners in the United Kingdom.' *Sociology of Health and Illness 28,* 7, 927–950.

Jones, L. and Fisher, T. (2006) 'Workforce trends in general practice: results from a longitudinal study of doctors' careers.' *British Journal of General practice 56,* 523, 134–136.

Klein, R. (1995) *The Politics of the NHS.* London: Longman.

Klein, R. (2007) 'Values Talk in the (English) NHS.' In S. Greer and D. Rowland (eds) *Devolving Policy, Diverging Values: The Values of the United Kingdom's National Health Services.* London: The Nuffield Trust.

Lester, H. and Roland, M. (2007) 'Future of quality measurement.' *British Medical Journal 335,* 7630, 1130–1131.

Lipsky, M. (1980) *Street-level Bureaucracy: Dilemmas of the Individual in Public Services.* New York: Russell.

Lupton, D. (1997) 'Doctors on the medical profession.' *Sociology of Health and Illness 19,* 4, 480–497.

Mangin, D. and Toop, L. (2007) 'The quality and outcomes framework. What have you done to yourselves?' *British Journal of General practice 57,* 539, 435–437.

McDonald, E.R. (2002) 'Street-level bureaucrats? Heart disease, health economics and policy in a primary care group.' *Health and Social Care in the Community 10,* 3, 129–135.

McDonald, M., Harrison, S., Checkland, K., Campbell, S.M. and Roland, M. (2007) 'Impact of financial incentives on clinical autonomy and internal motivation in primary care: an ethnographic study.' *British Medical Journal 334,* 7608, 1357–1359.

Pattison, S. (2004) 'Understanding Values.' In S. Pattison and R. Pill (eds) *Values in Professional Practice. Lessons for Health, Social Care and Other Professionals.* Oxford: Oxford University Press.

Pattison, S. and Pill, R. (eds) (2004) *Values in Professional Practice.* Oxford: Radcliffe Publishing Ltd.

Pollock, A. (2006) 'Privatising primary care.' *British Journal of General practice 56,* 529, 565–566.

Pringle, M. (1998) *Primary Care: Core Values.* London: British Medical Journal Books.

Ranade, W. (1998) 'Reforming the British National Health Service: All Change, No Change?' In W. Ranade (ed.) *Markets and Health Care.* London: Longman.

Rosser, W.W. (2002) 'The decline of family medicine as a career choice.' *Canadian Medical Association Journal 1666,* 110, 1419–1420.

Royal College of General Practitioners (RCGP) (1972) *The Future General Practitioner – Learning and Teaching*. London: RCGP.

Royal College of General Practitioners (RCGP) (2001) *Valuing General practice. Joint Paper by the RCGP, GP Committee of the BMA and The NHS Alliance*. London: RCGP.

Royal College of General Practitioners (RCGP) (2004) *The Future of General practice. A Statement by the Royal College of General Practitioners*. London: RCGP.

Royal College of General Practitioners (RCGP) (2006) *Profile of UK General Practitioners*. London: RCGP.

Royal College of General Practitioners (RCGP) (2007) *The Future Direction of General practice – a Road Map*. London: RCGP.

Smith, L.F.P. and Morrisey, J.R. (1994) 'Ethical dilemmas for general practitioners under the new NHS contract.' *Journal of Medical Ethics 20*, 3, 175–180.

Smith, R. (2005) 'The private sector in the English NHS: from pariah to saviour in under a decade.' *Canadian Medical Association Journal 173*, 2, 273–274.

Stacey, M. (1988) *The Sociology of Health and Healing*. London: Unwin Hyman.

Tudor-Hart, J. (2006) *A Political Economy of Health Care: A Clinical Perspective*. Bristol: Policy Press.

Wilkin, D., Hallam, L., Leavey, R. and Metcalfe, D. (1987) *Anatomy of Urban General practice*. London: Tavistock.

Chapter 5

Values and Mental Health Nursing

Ben Hannigan

INTRODUCTION

In this chapter, I will examine changing values in mental health nursing via a reading of historical and contemporary documents that review the work of this occupational group. I draw on three key sources, each endorsed by the United Kingdom government of the time, and each of which sets out recommendations for the future.

I write as an 'insider'; I trained and practised as a mental health nurse, and now teach and research in this area. For the benefit of readers unfamiliar with this world (which, I suggest, is very different from that of general, adult, nursing) I begin with some orienting observations on the origins and growth of this field of practice. I also contextualize my documentary examination throughout.

Using 'official', government-endorsed documents as the prism through which to view the work and values of an occupational group is a strategy that needs defending. Documents concerned with professional roles (including those authored at the request of, or for, government policymakers, along with those produced by, or for, professional associations and similar) can tell us something about the current status and anticipated future direction of a group. They may also reveal important data about an occupational group's place in a shifting division of labour, and say something about future aspirations. However, the relationship between reports and the real world of practice may be complex and tenuous. In and of themselves, documents may tell us little about what is happening in the workplace, including the content of practitioners' work and the values that may inform this. Practitioners and scholars concerned with these matters may, therefore, need to supplement their documentary analyses with (for example) observational and related research strategies.

Chapter 1 in this book makes clear the dynamic character of the world of health care work. Given this background of ongoing change, an important task in analysing reports centring on professional groups is to reflect on the specific contexts in which they are commissioned and produced. It is important, too, to consider the timing of reviews, and the ways in which evidence and opinion are gathered. Whilst change is ever-present, reports are, perhaps, likely to be produced during periods of particularly heightened occupational uncertainty, or in circumstances characterized by pressing wider social, political or other upheaval.

SOME ORIENTATING OBSERVATIONS[1]

The large-scale programme of asylum building in the United Kingdom (and elsewhere in the industrializing world) in the second half of the nineteenth century meant that hospitals were for many years the sole site of practice for those involved in the care of the mentally ill. With its roots in the asylum system, mental health nursing has a social history quite unlike that of general nursing. Over the years, men and women paid to look after people with mental health problems have laboured under a variety of titles. Before 'nurses' came 'asylum attendants', many of whom were working-class men valued for their physical strength (Dingwall, Rafferty and Webster 1988) and 'commonly regarded as the "unemployed of other professions"' (Nolan 1993, p.48). Like hospital-based nurses now, these workers had the greatest contact with patients. It was, however, medical practitioners who emerged as the most powerful group in the mental health field. Underpinning psychiatrists' claims to control the asylums was their successful advancement of the idea that mental illness was a disease with biophysical origins (Scull 1979).

Everyday asylum work initially required no formal preparation. The first training programme (the 'Certificate in Nursing the Insane') only appeared at the end of the nineteenth century (Nolan 1993). As

---

1   Parts of this section draw on material first published in Hannigan and Allen 2006.

psychiatric technologies advanced – exemplified by the use of physical treatments involving electricity, surgery and drugs (Prior 1993) – demand grew for a nursing workforce better equipped to undertake new tasks (Dingwall *et al.* 1988). Which body had the proper authority to specify the content of mental nurse training, and to license practitioners in this field, was hotly disputed. On one side was the Medico-Psychological Association (the precursor to today's Royal College of Psychiatrists, and the body responsible for the 'Certificate' referred to above), and on the other the General Nursing Council (GNC), which from 1919 had the responsibility to maintain a register of nurses (Dingwall *et al.* 1988). Rival training schemes overseen by these two organizations persisted into the early 1950s, until the (by then prefixed with the title 'Royal') Medico-Psychological Association finally agreed to discontinue its programme (Chatterton 2004).

By the middle of the twentieth century, then, nurses working in the mental health field could point to their programmes of preparation, instruction manuals and state registration as evidence of a growing professional status. Developments were also taking place in the world of knowledge. From the United States came the idea of nursing as a therapeutic, interpersonal activity (Peplau 1952). Whilst nurses in the UK tended to be less theoretically inclined than their North American counterparts, via the mediating influence of UK-based mental health nurse scholars such as Annie Altschul (Altschul 1972), the idea of an independent nursing function began to gain ground (Tilley 1999).

The social and political upheavals of the immediate post-World War II decades were significant for the shape of mental health services, and provide the larger backdrop to the first 'official' report into mental health nursing considered in this chapter. From the 1950s onwards community care emerged as an alternative to care in institutions. This international shift away from hospitals was driven by a combination of forces (Goodwin 1997). The economics of service provision were one important factor, with deinstitutionalization promising savings compared with expensive hospital care (Scull 1984). New medications enabled people with severe mental illnesses such as schizophrenia to gain respite from their often-distressing disturbances in thinking and perception. Significant, too, were wider social and cultural changes, reflected in ideological developments within the mental health field. Post-war social psychiatry, for example, emphasized environmental and interpersonal therapies in addition to physical treatments, whilst therapeutic communities questioned the idea of hierarchically organized hospitals. Goodwin (1997) points, too, to the ideological impact of the 'anti-psychiatry' movement, an increasing public tolerance of the presence of people with mental health problems living in community settings, and a growing service-user voice lobbying for community rather than institutional care. For mental health nurses, these challenges to institutional care manifested in new opportunities to practise beyond the walls of the asylum. 'Open door' policies appeared at pioneering hospitals (Nolan 2003), and nurses began the work of visiting patients and their families in their own homes. In the mid-1950s at Moorhaven Hospital in Devon, for example, nurses were specifically encouraged to develop therapeutic relationships with both patients and their relatives (Hunter 1974).

PSYCHIATRIC NURSING: TODAY AND TOMORROW

By the middle of the 1960s, then, much had changed in the world of mental health care. Nurses had made advances in their professional standing, and progress had been made in the generation of an independent knowledge base to underpin nursing work. Driven by wider social, political and ideological forces, change was also taking place in the sites of practice, with community care emerging (albeit on a small scale) as an alternative to hospital care. Until the mid-1960s, however, no formal review had been commissioned into the function and future of mental health nursing. Holding the first of its 22 meetings in 1965, the review team that went on to produce *Psychiatric Nursing: Today and Tomorrow* took its brief from two Ministry of Health committees to:

> consider the functions of psychiatric nursing staff and having regard to the changing pattern of psychiatric treatment to make recommendations, in the first instance on nursing staff patterns in wards and departments of hospitals for the mentally ill and psychiatric units in general hospitals. (Ministry of Health 1968, p.1)

Given the magnitude of the changes taking place in the mental health world at that time, the remit of the psychiatric nursing review team as reproduced above looks remarkably narrow in scope. Reflecting the status of nursing *vis-à-vis* medicine, the committee's deliberations were chaired by a senior psychiatrist, D.H. Clark, who later wrote an influential book on social therapy (Clark 1974). Nowadays, authors of reports aimed at the development of public services and the professions (including the authors of the two, later, mental health nursing reviews considered further in this chapter) are obliged to cast a wide net to gather evidence, and to consult with multiple representatives of interested parties. In contrast, the psychiatric nursing committee looked largely to its own resources, believing that whilst:

> [t]here was scope for substantial studies involving social scientists in the analysis and assessment of the actual work of nurses and their staffing patterns and possibly in attitude surveys...we were by no means sure that all the facts and figures so laboriously collected would add much to what we already knew or had learned from studies already available. (Ministry of Health 1968, p.2)

Read with contemporary eyes, this decision to favour anecdotal, 'insider', evidence over evidence scrupulously gathered through purposeful enquiry or wide consultation looks curious. 'Outsider' investigations conducted in the 1960s into the world of mental health care had tended to be critical of everyday, institutional, working practices (for example, see Goffman 1961). It seems plausible that by pooling their experiences and undertaking limited site visits, then, committee members may have been informed by a desire to protect their field from the possibility of further, unfavourable, examination.

Of those who gave evidence to the committee most were psychiatrists, some influential in their fields (including Russell Barton, who had earlier written *Institutional Neurosis* (Barton 1976), and Maxwell Jones, who was prominent in the therapeutic communities movement). All were described as practitioners with particular interests in nursing. Reflecting the narrowness of its brief, the psychiatric nursing review team in its final report limited itself to an account of recent developments in psychiatry and in psychiatric nursing, largely as these were practised in hospital settings. Care in the community, then emergent, warranted scant attention; this looks now like a major omission.

With a 'values' perspective in mind there is, though, content of great interest. As I have already noted, at the time when *Psychiatric Nursing: Today and Tomorrow* was commissioned, the idea of an independent, therapeutic, nursing function manifesting through the everyday interactions between practitioners and patients was developing. In a report otherwise notable for its emphasis on administrative matters it is significant that some, albeit passing, reference is made to the potential of nursing in this regard. Reflecting, perhaps, the professional interests of the psychiatrists consulted in the course of the review, this independent nursing role is particularly highlighted in the context of care in therapeutic communities and in the provision of social therapy. With respect to the development of nursing as an independent profession, however, the report offers little support for autonomous psychotherapeutic or socio-therapeutic practice, with any expansion of nursing roles being largely as a supportive adjunct to medicine.

Forty years on, *Psychiatric Nursing* appears to lack boldness, or a sense of connection with its wider context. Little evidence can be found that the turbulence surrounding the mental health world influenced the committee's thinking. Whilst considerable attention is paid to the administration of nursing – workforce numbers, hierarchies, the staffing of hospitals – little is paid to the principles underpinning mental health nursing practice, or to the wider challenges and opportunities facing mental health services. Recommendations for the future are tucked away at the report's end, and read as an afterthought. So far as it is now possible to tell, contemporary reactions to the publication of the report were muted. Commentaries were published in the *Nursing Mirror and Midwives Journal* and in the *Nursing Times*. In Nolan's authoritative history of mental health nursing, the review warrants only brief mention (Nolan 1993). For most nurses now, the document's existence is known only in so far as it is referred to in the preamble to the report which succeeded it – *Working in Partnership: A Collaborative Approach to Care* (Department of Health 1994).

For present purposes, however, *Psychiatric Nursing* stands as an important milestone. It remains the first (and, for over a quarter of a century, the only) review commissioned and sanctioned by a UK government into the work of mental health nurses. In having little to say about nursing values or the purposeful development of nursing practice, the report also serves as a revealing benchmark against which the two later reviews considered below might be compared.

WORKING IN PARTNERSHIP: A COLLABORATIVE APPROACH TO CARE

Following the publication of *Psychiatric Nursing: Today and Tomorrow* in 1968, 26 years passed before a successor review appeared. The intervening years were hardly uneventful. Both the scope and the scale of mental health services expanded during the 1970s and 1980s. Community care became a major enterprise, driven in part by large-scale policy initiatives such as *Better Services for the Mentally Ill* (Department of Health and Social Security 1975). Mental health nurses, whilst retaining their historic base in psychiatric hospitals, were increasingly found as core members of local, interprofessional, community mental health teams. Significant developments were also taking place in nursing practice, research and education. Mental health nurses were beginning to produce original research studies examining their work and function (for example, see Sladden 1979). In a practitioner discipline with, at that time, a still under-developed research base, in a landmark study Isaac Marks (a psychiatrist) demonstrated the effectiveness of mental health nurses in treating patients using behavioural methods (Marks 1985). From this grew a stream of projects investigating the effectiveness of nurses in treating specific mental illnesses (for example, see Brooker *et al.* 1994; Gournay and Brooking 1994). In the field of education, person-centred ideas were gaining particular ground, eventually being incorporated into England and Wales' 1982 syllabus for mental health nurse training (English and Welsh National Boards 1982).

Mental health services in the early 1990s – the period when work began on the production of *Working in Partnership* – were also facing a combination of distinct challenges. In many parts of the UK institutional care continued to be provided in outmoded, poorly equipped hospitals, often built in Victorian times. Community care, although firmly established, was chronically under-funded (Audit Commission 1994). Public and policymaking concerns, often widely reported by a critical media, centred on the apparent difficulties faced by organizations and workers in managing the risk of people with mental health problems harming either themselves or others (Hallam 2002).

Within the field of mental health nursing different 'camps' had emerged, associated with divergent, polarized, positions on nursing principles and practices (Burnard and Hannigan 2000). For example, drawing directly on ideas associated in an earlier era with Peplau

(Peplau 1952) and Altschul (Altschul 1972), Phil Barker (the UK's first professor of mental health nursing, based at Newcastle University) was arguing strongly for an independent, interpersonally mediated, role for nurses (Barker, Reynolds and Stevenson 1997). Championing a very different type of nursing was Kevin Gournay of London University's Institute of Psychiatry, who – with a personal practitioner background as a behavioural therapist – was pursuing the case for evidence-based mental health care delivered by practitioners of any stripe (Gournay 2001).

In the context of a wide-ranging review of all aspects of mental health policy and practice, the production of *Working in Partnership* was commissioned by the Secretary of State for Health, Virginia Bottomley. Mental health nursing by the early 1990s had matured sufficiently as a profession to include in its ranks a small number of senior academics, Barker and Gournay included; Tony Butterworth, a Manchester University professor with a background in community mental health nursing, was invited to chair a review team given the remit: '[t]o identify the future requirements for skilled nursing care in the light of developments in the provision of services for people with mental illness' (Department of Health 1994, p.vi).

Review team membership included nurses with roles in practice, education, research and management, along with representatives of other disciplines and users of mental health services. Subgroups were formed to pursue particular areas of work. Visits to services took place, and written and oral evidence was received from a large number of individuals and organizations.

Working in Partnership is an altogether more trenchant, action-oriented document than its predecessor, and is also broader in scope. It makes its case for the particular contribution of nurses to the mental health field based on practitioners' closeness to users of services and the value of the therapeutic nurse–patient relationship. Significant, too, is the report team's attempt to grapple with the core knowledge and skills of mental health nursing (and to a lesser extent, its values), and to make recommendations for necessary change.

Like *Psychiatric Nursing, Working in Partnership* opens with an account of the review body's methods of working. However, there is a marked contrast between the two reports, with the *Working in Partnership* team demonstrating its clear interest in consulting widely in the course of its deliberations. In the final document, reference is first made to background and context, before the expectations of nurses, their practice, patterns of service delivery, future challenges, and issues in research and education are addressed. The final report also includes 42 recommendations, each laid out at the document's end with key bodies to lead the process of implementation identified. The large number of recommendations (many of which had implications for mental health services in general, and for funding) suggests that the review team were of the view that significant action was needed to strengthen the nursing contribution to the provision of care.

For readers searching for continuity across reviews, and for evidence of the sustained value that mental health nurses place on the interpersonal, it is of interest to note that at the start of their report the *Working in Partnership* team declared its 'belief that the work of mental health nurses rests on their relationship with people who use mental health services' (Department of Health 1994, p.9). In addition, *Working in Partnership* challenged the profession to 're-examine every aspect of its policy and practice in the light of the needs of people who use services' (Department of Health 1994, p.5).

At the time of *Working in Partnership*'s publication, a common criticism was that many nurses lacked the practical ability to provide effective care and treatment for people with severe mental health problems such as schizophrenia (White 1993). In this context part of the review team's 're-examination' involved focusing very clearly on the skills expected of mental health nurses in the future. Core 'nursing skills' are, literally, listed in an appendix to the main document. 'Values' get a mention, too, but are not considered in such a systematic way. Thus it is (tantalizingly) stated that 'it is the combination of these particular skills, together with the values and practice common to the nursing profession as a whole, which provides the unique expertise of mental health nurses...' (Department of Health 1994, p.17).

Review team members – including its chair, Tony Butterworth – worked hard to raise the profile of their report and to lodge it firmly on to the profession's (and policymakers') agenda (see, for example, Butterworth 1994; Butterworth and Rushforth 1995). However, soon after the document's appearance it was reported in *The Guardian* newspaper that the likely cost of implementing the recommendations in full made them immediately unattractive to ministers: '[a]lthough Virginia Bottomley...has declared that mental health services must be given priority this year, she gave only lukewarm endorsement to the report of a review team she set up two years ago' (Brindle 1994, p.11).

Working in Partnership nonetheless had an impact on mental health nursing practice; or, perhaps more accurately, proved to be one force amongst a number contributing to change. One of the review team's better-remembered (and often invoked) key recommendations, for example, was that 'The essential focus for the work of mental health nurses lies in working with people with serious or enduring mental illness in secondary and tertiary care, regardless of setting' (Department of Health 1994, p.16). This proved a significant, and influential, statement, appearing as it did at a time when concerns were being raised that mental health nurses (particularly those working in the community) were providing the 'wrong type of care' (i.e. care that lacked an evidence base) for the 'wrong type of patients' (those with relatively transient, if still distressing, psychosocial problems) (Gournay 1994).

Overall, *Working in Partnership* reads as a far more professionally mature document than its predecessor. It celebrates the independent value of mental health nursing, but is also reflective and critical where necessary. Whilst an explicit language of 'values' is not used – with a language of 'skills' predominating – the document clearly pins the practice of mental health nurses on their pursuit of collaborative relationships with the people who use their services.

FROM VALUES TO ACTION

In comparison with the passing of more than a quarter of a century between the publication of *Psychiatric Nursing* and *Working in Partnership*, the final report considered here – *From Values to Action* (Department of Health 2006a) – appeared only 12 years after its predecessor. Commissioned by the Department of Health's Chief Nursing Officer, this new (and in an age of devolved government, England-only) review set out to answer the question: 'How can mental health nursing best contribute to the care of service users in the future?' (Department of Health 2006a, p.3).

This gap of scarcely more than a decade between root-and-branch occupational reviews is telling, and suggests a context of rapid policy and practice change, and an attendant uncertainty over roles and responsibilities in the mental health workplace. Policy activity in the mental health sphere has indeed been frenetic since the election of a 'modernizing' New Labour government in 1997 (6 and Peck 2004). New types of mental health team have appeared, and explicit action has been taken to break down professional boundaries. In this context other occupational groups, in addition to nursing, have been subject to government-inspired reviews of their work and future contribution. Reviews have, for example, been conducted into the work of psychiatrists in England (Department of Health 2005a), and both mental health nurses (Scottish Executive 2006a), and social workers (Scottish Executive 2006b), in Scotland.

The announcement of the plan to undertake this most recent review of mental health nursing was not universally well-received within the field. Writing in *The Guardian*, Phil Barker criticized the review process for being led by mandarins at the Department of Health rather than being conducted by representatives of nursing organizations independent of government (Barker 2005). Anecdotal evidence also suggests that not all were happy with the structure of the consultation process, which involved interested parties being invited to respond to carefully predetermined questions (Department of Health 2005b) rather than contributing free-flowing analyses of the state of the profession and the challenges ahead. Nonetheless, and in contrast to the inward-looking process through which (for example) *Psychiatric Nursing* was produced, representatives of all of mental health nursing's major organized bodies (including the Royal College of Nursing, the Mental Health Nurses' Association and Mental Health Nurse Academics UK) contributed to the stakeholder consultation, a process chaired by the Department of Health's Director of Mental Health Nursing. Many individual contributions were also received, along with responses from representatives of service-providing and educational organizations, and bodies representing other professional groups, users of mental health services, and carers.

From Values to Action, unlike either of its predecessors, is supported by a number of additional documents, including a comprehensive literature review into the effectiveness of mental health nursing interventions and a report of service user and carer views. A further document supporting the main report is a 'toolkit' designed to be of practical use to local organizations aiming to implement specific recommendations (Department of Health 2006b). Both are interesting, the first in reflecting mental health nursing's professional development by acknowledging that there is, now, 'a literature' in the field warranting consultation, the toolkit in that it suggests the review team's desire for practical action to follow the production of its report and recommendations.

The main document makes for interesting reading from a values perspective – not least for the obvious reason that the word 'values' appears in the report's title. Although it is possible to identify the principles that the *Working in Partnership* team believed underpinned good mental health nursing practice (the pursuit of collaborative, therapeutic, relationships, in particular) these were not couched in an explicit language of values. *From Values to Action*, however, reflects something of a 'values turn' taking place within the mental health world (and, indeed, within the health and social care field more widely, as this book testifies). This 'values turn' in mental health is elsewhere revealed in, for example, The Sainsbury Century for Mental Health's 'values workbook' (Woodbridge and Fulford 2004), in research papers focusing on values in the mental health sphere (see, for example, Nolan *et al.* 2004), and in the inclusion of chapters on values-based practice in textbooks for student mental health nurses (see, for example, Cooper 2009).

Against this wider background, here is what the *From Values to Action* document has to say about the relationships between values and practice:

> Mental health nursing will be a profession based on a clear set of values that informs every aspect of practice. Mental health nurses (MHNs) will work in partnership with service users of all ages, their carers and other professionals to improve the service user's experience and outcomes of care. MHNs will value the aspirations of the service user, offer meaningful choice in evidence-based interventions and care, adopt a positive attitude to personal change and support social inclusion. They will actively engage in combating stigma and ensure that service users from disadvantaged groups receive a truly responsive and inclusive service. (Department of Health 2006a, p.8)

This appears at a later point:

> The values held by people who work in mental health services directly influence their practice. In this report, we seek to be explicit about identifying the key values and principles that

all MHNs could identify with and use as the framework for all their activities. These values will influence direct clinical care, training and, above all, relationships with service users, carers and families. (Department of Health 2006a, p.17)

Three 'recommended sets of values' are set out: recovery approach values and principles; valuing the principle of equality; and valuing the need for evidence-based practice. Here, reference to 'recovery values' reflects a new and growing interest in the idea of recovery as being more than the eradication of symptoms (see, for example, Repper and Perkins 2003). Latterly, 'recovery' has come to denote a broad approach to care that emphasizes the importance of inclusion, citizenship and choice. Recovery also refers to a particular way of engaging in professional practice. In *From Values to Action* the relationship between nurses and service users – already identified as key in *Working in Partnership* – becomes the means through which recovery can be promoted.

The second component of *From Values to Action*'s new values-based approach to mental health nursing practice relates to the pursuit of equality; this, too, represents a continuation from *Working in Partnership*, which also recognized the imperative that closer attention should be paid to the needs of all sections of the community, including women and people from minority ethnic groups. Given the expectation that health care provision be evidence-based – allied to the obligation felt by professional groups to articulate the benefits of their particular contributions – it is unsurprising that the final 'recommended set of values' for mental health nurses is that their work should be effective.

CONCLUSION

Changes from a variety of sources – social, technological, professional – have opened up opportunities, such that yesterday's 'attendants' (occupied largely with the control of asylum patients with minimal regard for therapy) have become today's nurses concerned with the promotion of helping relationships and recovery. It remains the case that the relationship between written documents advocating particular modes of practice and the real-life workplace is, however, a complicated one. Professional values emerge in complex, socially mediated, ways, and in response to multiple factors of which a single report may be but one. For those concerned with the transmission and moulding of values (including the authors of reports like *From Values to Action*), great care needs to be taken lest 'recommended values' end up no more than being 'framed and solemnly hung up on entrance and office walls – or, even worse perhaps, laminated and pushed into a drawer or wallet and allowed to moulder quietly' (Pattison and Pill 2004, p.197).

Notwithstanding this warning I choose to close on a note of optimism. Both *Working in Partnership* and, now, *From Values to Action* resonate by reinforcing embedded principles, rather than by artificially imposing new ideals more likely to suffer the fate of 'death by lamination' (Pattison and Pill 2004). Whilst the detail of *From Values to Action* will eventually fade (and, indeed, the document itself be superseded), its underlying message, emphasizing the significance of helping relationships and the possibilities of positive change, captures important and durable values widely espoused in the nursing field. That these values have an enduring quality reflects, too, the degree to which mental health nursing has grown more assured of its place and future in its wider field of practice.

RESPONSE
Bronwen Davies

There is much of value in this chapter, not least the fact that, by writing an account of the emerging values within mental health nursing, Hannigan asserts that it is valid for me to regard myself as a professional. This is something which has been questioned throughout my career, both explicitly and implicitly.

I will focus here on three of the themes identified. These are: the emergence of mental health nursing as a profession; the contested occupational boundaries with other professions; and the particular struggles in which mental health nurses in the UK are currently engaged in expressing their professional values.

Hannigan is right to note the difference between 'espoused' values expressed in documents and the 'actual' world of practice. It is a cliché within nursing that there is distrust of management and of academics: nursing is often characterized as essentially practical, 'hands on' work. Nurses who have moved into management or teaching – that is, those nurses most likely to develop and articulate professional standards and values – can be seen to have removed themselves from 'real' nursing. Their pronouncements, views and values can thus be derogated as unlikely to offer anything useful to 'real' nurses in their occupational lives.

Hannigan traces the development of mental health nursing as an occupational group over the past 50 years in the UK. This includes the years in which I have worked as a mental health nurse. This period is one in which mental health nursing has established itself as a profession. The distrust of mental health nurse managers and academics that has been evident at practitioner level may be characteristic of an emerging professional group that has not yet reached maturity, but that is still 'storming and norming', prior to 'performing' (see Tuckman 1965). I see some evidence recently of changing attitudes in this respect.

Hannigan notes that medical practitioners emerged as the most powerful group in the mental health field during the first half of the twentieth century, underpinned by the successful advancement of the idea that 'mental illness was a disease with biophysical origins'. The second half of the century has seen the advancement of the idea that the social understanding and treatment of illness is critical to the development of health care systems and to health improvement. Developing a social understanding of illness leads inevitably to questions about power and control, between citizens and health professionals, between patients and health professionals, and between different occupational groups. Mental health nursing is but one of a number of professions that have developed in the mental health field within this context, others being social work, clinical psychology and occupational therapy.

When *Psychiatric Nursing: Today and Tomorrow* (1968) was published, it was thought proper that medical professionals should examine and define the scope and practice of nursing, something that would not occur today. However, mental health nursing has developed not only through a contested occupational boundary with psychiatry, but also through one with social work. By the time that *Working in Partnership* (1994) was produced, the State had laid the legislative groundwork for defining some of the care that patients receive after becoming ill as 'social' care; this has to be paid for, unlike health care which remains largely free under the NHS (Department of Health 1990). Social workers' role was to assess need and subsequently organize social care for individuals whose needs met local authority criteria. The care of individuals with a mental illness who did *not* need social care, or whose needs did *not* meet local authority criteria, became the responsibility of health professionals. Because they are the largest professional group in the field, this work falls mainly to mental health nurses. In this context, the impact of *Working in Partnership* (1994) in promoting the values espoused by mental health nursing as a profession was considerable. Hannigan notes that it made 'a case for the particular contribution of nurses to the mental health field based on practitioners' closeness with users of services and their valuing of the therapeutic nurse/patient relationship'.

Exactly how nurses do this has been revealed increasingly in the professional literature since that time. One of the review's recommendations was that mental health nurses no longer called themselves 'psychiatric nurses', implying an occupation practising within the medical model of health and illness. Calling ourselves 'mental health nurses' intentionally defines our professional practice as lying within a social context, in which good health is promoted even for those living with a chronic mental illness. By doing this, mental health nurses were not only emancipating themselves from control by psychiatrists, but also asserting that emancipation to social workers.

Developments in sociological and psychological understanding of mental illness, together with economic pressures, have led the move away from hospital-based care and rooted treatment and care of mental illness into 'community' settings (clinics, health centres, homes, supported accommodation, leisure centres and other public places). At the same time, better understanding about the biophysical changes that take place in those with a mental illness has contributed hugely to improvements in treatment and prognosis.

Attendants/nurses have always had more continuous close contact with patients than medical practitioners. While clinics and ward rounds are the settings in which patients are presented to medical practitioners, either of their own accord or by nurses, it is the ward itself, the patient's home, the clinic and other community settings that are the sites of nursing work. Hannigan notes that, during the 1970s and 1980s, mental health nurses were increasingly found 'as core members of local, interprofessional community mental health teams'. It is my observation that, although government documents assume that the community mental health team (CMHT) is the form through which mental health care is organized and delivered in the UK, it is far from the case that all CMHTs include professions other than mental health nurses as core members. Psychiatrists, social workers, occupational therapists and clinical psychologists should all be found in the model CMHT, but commonly these professionals have responsibilities to several teams or departments and only work part-time in a CMHT. It might be more accurate to recognize that CMHTs, like ward teams in a hospital, are first and foremost nursing teams with access to consultation with other professionals that varies, in quantity and quality, between localities.

In my experience, considerable work took place within the profession in response to *Working in Partnership* (1994), laying the groundwork for the production of *From Values to Action* (2006). This explicitly set out three 'sets of values' for mental health nurses, namely: valuing the principles of the recovery approach; valuing the principle of equality; and valuing the need for evidence-based practice. Valuing the principles of the recovery approach places mental health nursing practice very firmly within a social model of health and illness. Within this model the medical focus on alleviating distressing symptoms, primarily through pharmaceutical intervention, plays a necessary but not sufficient part in the care and treatment of those with mental illness. Once it is acknowledged that the environment of care and psychologically based interventions both have a role to play in both producing and alleviating symptoms, the decision as to which type or combination of interventions is the best for a particular individual at a particular time can only be decided by sharing professional knowledge and skills. For this reason I believe mental health nurses and psychiatrists should work closely with each other, as well as with service users and their families/carers.

I entered mental health nursing before it was recognized as professional work, bringing with me the greatest respect for the skills of mental health nurses whom I knew and for the empathy and compassion they displayed in their everyday work with patients. It has been heartening to see the work of mental health nurses increasingly recognized over recent years, and also to see the values of mental health nursing increasingly articulated. Mental health nurses still step back, at times, from asserting their professional knowledge, leaving key decisions about patient care to psychiatrists or social workers. At other times, however, mental health nurses are making key decisions, with patients, about appropriate care and treatment, are enacting these plans and are happy to be accountable for their practice. The legislative principles embodied in the Mental Health Act (2008) give mental health nurses a framework to further develop as a profession and take forward the values of respect for difference, working in partnership and improving the health of those with mental illness.

REFERENCES

6, P. and Peck, E. (2004) 'New Labour's modernization in the public sector: a neo-Durkheimian approach and the case of mental health services.' *Public Administration 82*, 1, 83–108.

Altschul, A. (1972) *Patient-nurse Interaction: A Study of Interaction Patterns in Acute Psychiatric Wards.* Edinburgh: Churchill Livingstone.

Audit Commission (1994) *Finding a Place: A Review of Mental Health Services for Adults.* London: HMSO.

Barker, P. (2005) 'Caring about caring.' *The Guardian*, 27 April.

Barker, P., Reynolds, W. and Stevenson, C. (1997) 'The human science basis of psychiatric nursing: theory and practice.' *Journal of Advanced Nursing 25*, 4, 660–667.

Barton, R. (1976) *Institutional Neurosis* (3rd edn). Bristol: John Wright and Sons.

Brindle, D. (1994) 'Bottomley cool on mental health report: Minister keeps distance from review team's proposals.' *The Guardian*, 11 March.

Brooker, C., Falloon, I., Butterworth, A., Goldberg, D., Graham-Hole, V. and Hillier, V. (1994) 'The outcome of training community psychiatric nurses to deliver psychosocial intervention.' *British Journal of Psychiatry 165*, 2, 222–230.

Burnard, P. and Hannigan, B. (2000) 'Qualitative and quantitative approaches in mental health nursing: moving the debate forward.' *Journal of Psychiatric and Mental Health Nursing 7*, 1, 1–6.

Butterworth, T. (1994) 'Working in partnership: a collaborative approach to care. The review of mental health nursing.' *Journal of Psychiatric and Mental Health Nursing 1*, 1, 41–44.

Butterworth, T. and Rushforth, D. (1995) 'Working in partnership with people who use services: reaffirming the foundations of practice for mental health nursing.' *International Journal of Nursing Studies 32*, 4, 373–385.

Chatterton, C. (2004) '"Caught in the middle"? Mental nurse training in England 1919–51.' *Journal of Psychiatric and Mental Health Nursing 11*, 1, 30–35.

Clark, D.H. (1974) *Social Therapy in Psychiatry.* Harmondsworth: Penguin.

Cooper, L. (2009) 'Values Based Mental Health Nursing Practice.' In P. Callaghan, J. Playle and L. Cooper (eds) *Mental Health Nursing Skills.* Oxford: Oxford University Press.

Department of Health (1990) *NHS and Community Care Act.* London: HMSO.

Department of Health (1994) *Working in Partnership: A Collaborative Approach to Care: Report of the Mental Health Nursing Review Team.* London: Department of Health.

Department of Health (2005a) *New Ways of Working for Psychiatrists: Enhancing Effective, Person-centred Services through New Ways of Working in Multidisciplinary and Multi-agency Contexts. Final report 'But Not the End of the Story'.* London: Department of Health.

Department of Health (2005b) *Chief Nursing Officer's Review of Mental Health Nursing: Consultation Document.* London: Department of Health.

Department of Health (2006a) *From Values to Action: The Chief Nursing Officer's Review of Mental Health Nursing.* London: Department of Health.

Department of Health (2006b) *Self-assessment Toolkit. From Values to Action: The Chief Nursing Officer's Review of Mental Health Nursing.* London: Department of Health.

Department of Health and Social Security (1975) *Better Services for the Mentally Ill.* London: HMSO.

Dingwall, R., Rafferty, A.M. and Webster, C. (1988) *An Introduction to the Social History of Nursing.* London: Routledge.

English and Welsh National Boards (1982) *Syllabus of Training: Professional Register Part 3 (Registered Mental Nurse).* London: English and Welsh National Boards for Nursing, Midwifery and Health Visiting.

Goffman, E. (1961) *Asylums.* Harmondsworth: Penguin.

Goodwin, S. (1997) *Comparative Mental Health Policy: From Institutional to Community Care.* London: Sage.

Gournay, K. (1994) 'Redirecting the emphasis to serious mental illness.' *Nursing Times 90*, 25, 40–41.

Gournay, K. (2001) 'Guest editorial. Mental health nursing in 2001: what happens next?' *Journal of Psychiatric and Mental Health Nursing 8*, 6, 473–476.

Gournay, K. and Brooking, J. (1994) 'Community psychiatric nurses in primary health care.' *British Journal of Psychiatry 165,* 2, 231–238.

Hallam, A. (2002) 'Media influences on mental health policy: long-term effects of the Clunis and Silcock cases.' *International Review of Psychiatry 14,* 1, 26–33.

Hannigan, B. and Allen, D. (2006) 'Complexity and change in the United Kingdom's system of mental health care.' *Social Theory & Health 4,* 3, 244–263.

Hunter, P. (1974) 'Community psychiatric nursing in Britain: an historical review.' *International Journal of Nursing Studies 11,* 4, 223–233.

Marks, I. (1985) 'Controlled trial of psychiatric nurse therapists in primary care.' *British Medical Journal 290,* 6476, 1181–1184.

Ministry of Health (1968) *Psychiatric Nursing: Today and Tomorrow.* London: HMSO.

Nolan, P. (1993) *A History of Mental Health Nursing.* London: Chapman and Hall.

Nolan, P. (2003) 'The History of Community Mental Health Nursing.' In B. Hannigan and M. Coffey (eds) *The Handbook of Community Mental Health Nursing.* London: Routledge.

Nolan, P., Haque, M.S., Bourke, P. and Dyke, R. (2004) 'A comparison of the work and values of community mental health nurses in two mental health NHS Trusts.' *Journal of Psychiatric and Mental Health Nursing 11,* 5, 525–533.

Pattison, S. and Pill, R. (2004) 'Professions and values: a dynamic relationship.' In S. Pattison and R. Pill (eds) *Values in Professional Practice: Lessons for Health, Social Care and Other Professionals.* Oxford: Radcliffe Medical Press.

Peplau, H. (1952) *Interpersonal Relations in Nursing.* New York: G.P. Putnam and Sons.

Prior, L. (1993) *The Social Organization of Mental Illness.* London: Sage.

Repper, J. and Perkins, R. (2003) *Social Inclusion and Recovery: A Model for Mental Health Practice.* Edinburgh: Baillière Tindall.

Scottish Executive (2006a) *Rights, Relationships and Recovery: The Report of the National Review of Mental Health Nursing in Scotland.* Edinburgh: Scottish Executive.

Scottish Executive (2006b) *Changing Lives: Report of the 21st Century Social Work Review.* Edinburgh: Scottish Executive.

Scull, A. (1979) *Museums of Madness: The Social Organization of Insanity in Nineteenth-century England.* London: Allen Lane.

Scull, A. (1984) *Decarceration: Community Treatment and the Deviant: A Radical View* (2nd edn). Cambridge: Polity Press.

Sladden, S. (1979) *Psychiatric Nursing in the Community: A Study of a Working Situation.* Edinburgh: Churchill Livingstone.

Tilley, S. (1999) 'Altschul's legacy in mediating British and American psychiatric nursing discourses: common sense and the "absence" of the accountable practitioner.' *Journal of Psychiatric and Mental Health Nursing 6,* 4, 283–295.

Tuckman, B.W. (1965) 'Developmental sequence in small groups.' *Psychological Bulletin 63,* 6, 384–399.

White, E. (1993) 'Community Psychiatric Nursing 1980 to 1990: A Review of Organization, Education and Practice.' In C. Brooker and E. White (eds) *Community Psychiatric Nursing: A Research Perspective, Volume 2.* London: Chapman and Hall.

Woodbridge, K. and Fulford, K.W.M. (2004) *Whose Values? A Workbook for Values-based Practice in Mental Health Care.* London: The Sainsbury Centre for Mental Health.

Chapter 6

Values and Adult General Nursing

Derek Sellman

INTRODUCTION

It might be supposed that the values of nursing in general, and of adult nursing in particular, are sufficiently understood to make the exercise of articulating those values unnecessary. Thus it would be uncontroversial to suggest that nurses should, for example, be caring, compassionate and trustworthy. That these expectations hold sway is evidenced by reactions to incidents in which nurses are found to have acted in ways contrary to these values. The nurse who deliberately ended the life of several older persons in his care by the administration of insulin,[1] and the nurse who injected patients in an accident and emergency department to cause life-threatening episodes,[2] both earn our censure precisely because they abuse the position of trust that comes with being a registered nurse. Hence there is a sense in which the core values of nursing have remained consistent since Florence Nightingale (and others) managed to change public perception of nurses from the Sairey Gamp image evoked by Charles Dickens in *Martin Chuzzlewit*, to that of a suitable occupation for ladies of good character.[3]

---

1   In March 2008 Colin Norris began a 30-year jail sentence for the murder of four elderly patients in his care during a six-month period in 2002.

2   In May 2006 Benjamin Geen was given 17 life sentences for the murder of two patients and for grievous bodily harm to 15 others during a nine-week period between December 2003 and February 2004 by injecting various drugs to induce respiratory arrest in those patients in the accident and emergency department in which he worked as a staff nurse.

3   Although the description of nurses as 'grubby, drunken and promiscuous' by Lord Mancroft in the House of Lords in February 2008, after he had recently been a patient in a Bath hospital, might lead some to believe that the descendants of Sairey Gamp are alive, well and among us still.

Nightingale's accomplishments have been somewhat overlooked as her reputation for requiring discipline and obedience above all else in her probationers has grown out of all proportion to her influence on modern nursing. I have outlined elsewhere how Nightingale's requirement for obedience has been misinterpreted because of the limited vision of many of her followers, and argued that a more measured review of her influence would rehabilitate her reputation (Sellman 1997). Suffice it to say here that hers was not a call for blind unthinking obedience, but a requirement (appropriate to the social *mores* of the times) for conformity with the orders of those with purported greater knowledge, *and only in so far as those orders were based on accurate observation, proper reason and a respectful regard for the wellbeing of patients.* Regardless of her tarnished reputation, the core values of nursing still promulgated as appropriate for nursing and nurse in the early part of the twenty-first century can be traced back to Nightingale and others (including Mary Seacole). Were she to read the current UK code for nurses (NMC 2008), Nightingale might be surprised by the emphasis on personal autonomy, but she would recognize the consistency of many of the injunctions with her own view of the values important for nurses.

Since the 1970s these core values have been increasingly subjected to challenge because of a rise in the volume and frequency of significant changes in the ways nursing is organized, delivered and monitored. Before the 1970s, in most instances major change to the provision of health services in the UK was instituted only after a lengthy period of review, consultation and planning. A Royal Commission (which would take months, if not years, to complete) was seen as the standard by which this process should proceed; the implementation of (selected) recommendations of the final report would include efforts to minimize disruption. Change under these circumstances would, in general terms, follow Lewin's (1951) model of moving from a stable, but unsatisfactory state, to a new, more desirable state, via a planned, and quite lengthy transition period. Change nowadays is endemic, with imperatives seeming to demand instant, short-term responses without space or opportunity for stabilization or effective evaluation before the next directives for change arrive. The constant sense of instability engendered can potentially increase resistance, with individuals suspecting that new sets of demands will arrive even before the current changes are completed, never mind established. Working in an unstable environment characterized by constant change adds to the already burdensome demands of nursing work created by its interface with human suffering and distress.

Nurses have been subjected to external imperatives in the same way, and to the same extent as other health and social care service-providers. Thus the underlying assumptions of a market-driven, resource-conscious health service have been adopted by nurses, particularly those given budgetary responsibility. But the imperatives have not only been external. The rise of the professional aspirations of nurses illustrated in the battle for professional autonomy[4] has only added internal pressures for change to the myriad externally imposed imperatives to which nurses have been required to respond.

The effect of all this change on the core values of nursing has yet to be the subject of major systematic or empirical enquiry. The aim of this chapter is to begin to articulate some of the ways in which it appears that modern imperatives have influenced the core values of nursing, in the hope that questions of an empirical nature might emerge. These might, in turn, indicate suitable empirical methods of investigation for this important area of professional work.

THE CORE VALUES OF NURSING

The core values of nursing are largely accepted as being unproblematic; they are related to general, but often unspecified, ideas of care, compassion and trustworthiness. It can be argued, however, that these long-held values are under threat from the influence of a set of more instrumental, managerial values whose emphasis on value for money, meeting targets, aiming for higher positions in league tables and so on, tends both to distort, and to change, the priorities of practices. Instrumental managerial values need not necessarily be inconsistent with the values of nursing; effective, caring service requires a bureaucracy, even if this bureaucracy is constrained by financial limitations (see Chapter 10 for a sustained development of this point). However, it is problematic if these instrumental values are allowed, either to corrupt the core values of nursing, or to become *the* values to which all other sets of values in the provision of health care are subordinated.

---

4   See, for example, the debates in the nursing press and beyond during the period leading to the publication of the first UK code of conduct for nurses in 1983.

This notion of corruption of values forms part of MacIntyre's (1985) critique of institutions. For MacIntyre, it is institutions' tendency to allow instrumental values to become dominant that poses the greatest danger to the practices that they exist to enable. Nursing requires some form of bureaucracy to function with any degree of organization or sense of purpose. However, the institutionalization tendencies of bureaucracies have, as Weber predicted (Gerth and Mills 1948, pp.196–244; see also Lassman 2000), continued to grow exponentially, leaving nursing and individual nurses struggling to balance the needs of, and for, economy with patients' care needs. Twenty-first century institutions in liberal democracies have developed some particularly demanding bureaucratic surveillance and control measures that impose restrictions on what practitioners can or cannot do, and that require resource intensive forms of accounting (Power 1997). These demands appear likely to increase despite periodic exhortations to 'cut red tape', or to adopt a 'light touch' in reviewing performance.

According to MacIntyre, the corrupting influence of institutions on practices is inevitable because the aims of the institutions are fundamentally at odds with the aims of practices. The resultant clash between what MacIntyre initially referred to as 'external goods' and 'internal goods' (1985, pp.181–204) and later termed 'goods of effectiveness' and 'goods of excellence' (1988, pp.31–46) reflects respectively the different values that underpin the different types of activities for which institutions and practices exist.

MACINTYRE'S NOTION OF PRACTICES

In his book *After Virtue*, Alasdair MacIntyre (1985) sets out his vision of a particular category of human activity: a type of activity in which it is possible for individuals to pursue excellences within a social and moral framework. He calls this type of activity a 'practice'. The term 'practice' denotes:

> ...any coherent and complex form of socially established cooperative human activity through which goods internal to that form of activity are realised in the course of trying to achieve those standards of excellence which are appropriate to, and partially definitive, of that form of activity... (MacIntyre 1985, p.187)

MacIntyre offers chess as a paradigm case here. In initiating a child into playing chess, it may at first be necessary to offer an inducement (he suggests sweets). But the child may soon learn that there is something in the game of chess that makes it desirable beyond the promise of sweets. If this happens, the child will have moved from playing chess for external reward (obtaining sweets) to engaging with chess for intrinsic reasons and satisfactions. This something *other than mere external reward* is what MacIntyre means by the 'goods internal to that form of activity', as outlined in his definition of a practice quoted above.

With the child's growing recognition of chess as a practice (i.e. a form of activity that provides access to a set of internal goods) comes the recognition that the internal goods are only accessible under certain conditions. MacIntyre sets out these conditions as a requirement for the core virtues of a practice: the virtue of justice, the virtue of courage and the virtue of honesty. Without these three virtues a practice may collapse into an activity that no longer offers access to a set of internal goods. It becomes fundamentally distorted.

For MacIntyre the virtues of honesty, courage and justice sustain the relationships between individuals engaged in the practice. It is the pursuit, or at least the acceptance, of these virtues that differentiates a practice from other forms of activity. For example, the internal goods of chess relate to playing the game well rather than (necessarily) to win: if winning, especially for reward or prizes, were to become the sole aim, then the temptation to win by cheating would probably exert a corrupting influence, particularly if the majority of chess players came to value winning more than playing well.

For 'playing well', 'excellence' might be substituted. This would be consistent with MacIntyre's choice of term; and striving for excellence in chess requires conformity to the standards by which excellence is judged by those already engaged in chess as a practice. In this sense, winning is consistent with chess as a practice only when a player wins by having played an excellent game: excellent both in terms of strategic moves and in terms of the pursuit of human excellences – that is, the virtues of honesty, courage and justice. To win by means contrary to these three virtues is to preclude access to the internal goods of the practice.

MacIntyre (1985, pp.181–204) points out that a practice will have both internal and external goods and that the balance between these goods is critical. A practice can only remain a practice while this balance favours the internal goods: in other words, while a majority of practitioners remain committed to the values of their practice, underpinned by a respect for the standards of excellence intrinsic to that practice. Should this balance be lost (as would be the case with chess if a majority played solely in pursuit of external reward) then the practice as a whole would be corrupted precisely because the adoption of a set of extrinsic instrumental values would undermine the pursuit of human excellences. From this, MacIntyre concludes that only a practice in good order can resist such corrupting influences. In other words, a practice is only sustainable in so far as its practitioners engage with it as a practice; this inevitably requires a commitment to the core virtues of honesty, courage and justice.

NURSING AS A MACINTYREAN PRACTICE

I have suggested elsewhere that nursing provides an opportunity for individuals to pursue a selection of internal goods and thus it is appropriate to consider nursing as a type of MacIntyrean practice (Sellman 2000). Understanding nursing thus as a practice acknowledges that to work as a nurse is to aspire to a particular set of intrinsic standards of excellence that help to define nursing as a practice; these include aspiring to the virtues of honesty, courage and justice. These virtues underpin the core values of nursing and they are reflected in much of what appears in the UK code for nurses (NMC 2008). On this account, nursing presents an occupation that has the potential to offer individuals something *other than mere external reward*: in other words, to engage with nursing as a practice is to gain access to internal and intrinsic, as well as to external and extrinsic, goods.

This idea of the existence of something other than mere external reward in nursing can be identified in much of the nursing literature, particularly in parts where representational models or theoretical constructs are considered in the context of defining the nature of nursing. It is also reflected in the abundant normative claims made by nurses and nursing scholars, for example:

- in the popular notion that nursing is more than a mere set of tasks to be performed in response to particular patient symptoms

- in the idea that nursing should offer a holistic approach to patient care on the grounds that health and illness has, amongst other things, physical, psychological, sociological, and spiritual origins and consequences

- in the demand for recognition of the unique contribution that nurses can make to the health and wellbeing of individuals and communities.

While many of these claims lack evidential substance, they point to a dissatisfaction (at least within nursing circles) with the way in which the purported difficult-to-articulate, but intrinsically important, aspects of nursing are marginalized in the current climate of evidence-based practice and the justificatory requirements it has engendered.

Partly in response to his critics, and partly to express his ideas with more clarity, MacIntyre (1988, pp.31–46) later uses the terms 'goods of effectiveness' and 'goods of excellence' to replace his earlier terms of 'external goods' and 'internal goods' respectively. The term 'goods of effectiveness' expresses the idea that it is the pursuit of such goods understood in purely instrumental terms that corrupts practices. And if there is a clash of values between extrinsically oriented institutions and intrinsically oriented practices, then the different understandings of evidence-based practice currently available provide an instantiation of where this tension is manifest.

THE RISE OF EVIDENCE-BASED PRACTICE

Notions of evidence-based practice (EBP) have permeated the full range of regulated health and social care professional activity wholesale (Rolfe, Segrott and Jordan 2008). However, the term is both wide-ranging and inconsistently interpreted. EBP is an idea to which both the institutions and the practices within health and social care can subscribe precisely because it seems to offer the promise of being compatible with the particular values of each. An institution[5] can adopt EBP because of its value in the pursuit of the goods of effectiveness. A practice can make a case for EBP as a way of pursuing the goods of excellence.

While there may be agreement between institutions and practices on the value of EBP, agreement on its meaning and purpose is less

---

5   Institution here should be understood in the way that MacIntyre uses the term. In this sense an institution is a bureaucratic entity that exerts a controlling and corrupting influence on a practice. Institutions can be virtual as well as physical – so regulatory bodies as well as hospitals or primary health care trusts would be institutions under this description.

forthcoming; each tends to be swayed by understandings that best fit with their respective values. The rhetoric surrounding the EBP movement can allow the institution to use it instrumentally as an addition to the armoury of measurement of value for money, performance indicators and so on; it may even be used as a means of curtailing expenditure implications of clinical decisions. By contrast, practices can adopt EBP both to find support for standards of excellence and as a way of justifying the need for additional resources if patients' and communities' needs are to be met. These different understandings reflect different conceptions of the nature of evidence.

For some, there is a clear understanding that the only data worthy of note is what is often referred to as 'hard evidence'. This is evidence derived from experimental quantitative studies in which the variables are controlled to the point at which the possibility of error is all but removed (see, for example, Paley 2006). In this context, the randomized controlled trial (RCT) functions as the 'gold standard' of research design, and validity is further enhanced by the adoption of systematic review and meta-analysis, the purpose of which is to compare findings from multiple RCT studies to reduce the possibility of error further. At the extreme in this schema, only quantitative studies get a foothold on the hierarchy of evidence in terms of contributing to systematic reviews or meta-analyses (see, for example, SIGN 2002). Exclusion of anything that lies outside the scientific method is at the heart of the meaning of evidence in this radical vision of EBP.

For others, evidence includes qualitative studies and allows for expert opinion and professional expertise (see, for example, Flemming and Fenton 2002). While rejecting the dominance of the narrow scientific method, many of those 'inclusionists' (Paley 2006) who hold with this expansion of the evidence base for EBP tend to argue for their position using the language of quantitative research. More precisely, they tend to adopt the requirements of quantitative research and argue for the need for a different set of measures to determine, for example, validity. So, the validity measures for qualitative research must be different from validity measures in quantitative research because the nature of the phenomena being studied is different. Paley (2006) problematizes this, pointing out that while quantitative research seeks to minimize the possibility of error using rigorous statistical methodology, qualitative studies tend to equate validity with high levels of consensus among particular communities – hardly equivalent levels of validity.

Nevertheless, inclusionists continue to argue that while quantitative research can be accepted as the 'gold standard' for measuring outcomes where interventions have been systematically controlled, it cannot offer insight into personal experience. Thus the hard facts of RCTs need to be complemented by findings from qualitative methods. Quantitative studies may provide the answers to questions about, for example, which drug(s) may work best for a given condition, or which proprietary dressing best promotes healing in specific types of wounds. But only qualitative studies can shed light on whether treatments add to patients' sense of wellbeing, comfort, or quality of life. Without qualitative research, the inclusionists argue, understandings of the human experience of health and illness are inadequate.

While the rhetoric of EBP continues unabated, significant tensions remain between those who claim it as the 'holy grail' of health and social care delivery and those who see it as but one among a number of sources of evidence.[6]

THE CLASH OF VALUES

If MacIntyre's schema is correct, EBP could be seen as an instrument of the institutions' single-minded pursuit of goods of effectiveness (at the expense of goods of excellence). It is a significant corrupting influence on the values of health and social care practices and practitioners. Its significance is perhaps all the more insidious given that practices themselves have adopted the rhetoric of evidence-based care. Practices cannot do otherwise, of course; to argue against the logic of EBP is to court accusations of charlatanism, and no professional practice would wish to marginalize itself in this way. Thus professional practices have to engage in the discussions about the purposes and meanings of EBP.

It is overly simplistic to state that the primary focus of nursing as a practice is to provide care, while the primary focus of the health care institution is to manage the delivery of that care within fixed budgets; but this does reflect something of the overall purpose of institutions and practices. This difference in outlook and fundamental values is not new.

---

6   The NMC (the UK professional and regulatory body for nursing) appears to want it both ways in requiring of nurses that: 'You must deliver care based on the best available evidence or best practice' (NMC 2008, p.7). The ambiguity of this statement seems lost on the NMC; it could be taken to mean either (a) that in the absence of available evidence then the nurse must deliver care based on best practice or (b) that the nurse can choose between either best available evidence or best practice in delivering care.

There have always been financial constraints placed upon health and social care practitioners. It was naïve when the NHS was founded in 1948 to assume that once existing needs were met, demands on the service would decrease when, in fact, there has been an inexorable increase. Thus contemporary practitioners cannot ignore issues of economy and resource allocation. But this should not necessarily compromise the core values of nursing: and probably few of those who represent the institutions would wish nursing to abandon the intrinsic 'ideal of service' (Sockett 1993, p.16) to which nurses continue to aspire.

However, despite the best efforts of those, such as managers, who represent institutions to mitigate the worst excesses of extrinsic policy dictate, the effectiveness orientation of institutions continues to chip away at the core values of nursing. This is insidious as nurses continually have to justify their contribution to patient care in ways determined by values external to the practice of nursing.

One widespread way in which institutional values can threaten or erode practice values comes from the ubiquitous requirement for effectiveness measurement couched in the form of crude indicators of performance, outcome or need. Because the things that nurses value most (things relating to intrinsic goods of excellence inherent in practice) are difficult to articulate or to measure easily (in terms that those pursuing instrumental effectiveness understand), existent measurement tools remain fixed in the domain of goods of effectiveness. Consequently the goods of excellence, while sometimes acknowledged as important by the instrumentalists, are obscured from view in the accounting. And effectively, 'If you can't count it, it doesn't count' (Handy 1996, p.137; also see Pattison 1997, pp.94–96). Thus intrinsic values of care in nursing are powerfully devalued.

Worryingly, perhaps, the divergence between institutions and practices seems to be widening as the institutions respond to the pull of political and financial targets while practices respond to the pull of the ideal of service; and the pull of each impacts upon the values both. According to MacIntyre (1985), practices must remain in good order if they are to resist the corrupting influence of the institutions; and he understands a practice in good order as one where those engaged with it strive towards the excellences that (at least partly) define it as a practice. Thus the practice of nursing (understood as an occupation that can offer something *other than mere external reward*) can continue only so long as the balance between internal goods and external goods either favours the former, or, at the very least, enables practitioners continuing access to those internal goods. Faced with the sometimes overwhelming pull of instrumental values from employing institutions, practitioners can adopt one of three general responses: wholesale adoption of instrumental values; wholesale rejection of instrumental values; or an attempt to accommodate instrumental values within a framework that values the goods of excellence.

To wholly adopt instrumental values would be to abandon nursing as a practice. The wholesale acceptance of nursing work as solely in the domain of goods of effectiveness is inimical to those features of nursing that involve care, compassion and trustworthiness. It risks placing the meeting of financial targets, scoring well on league tables, and maximizing the efficient use of resources above the needs of individual patients. This may well allow more patients to be processed in, for example, a chronic pain clinic, and help to ensure that no one client remains on the clinic waiting list for longer than whatever target time period has been externally determined as appropriate. But the specific needs of individual patients are likely not to be met. And, ironically, it may be that a failure to provide properly focused individual care and consultation may lead to more expense later on.

To reject instrumental values altogether is to refuse to justify actions in terms of external, extrinsic goods. It might involve individual practitioners doing such things as refusing to complete the myriad externally imposed forms used as purported measures or validations of performance, refusing to participate in burdensome review, or refusing to cooperate with externally imposed imperatives on the grounds that such activities detract from patient care. Time spent filling in forms is time unavailable for direct patient contact – a sentiment often heard from nurses. And most externally imposed demands and changes lack the kind of evidence base that these same instrumentalists demand from practitioners to justify clinical actions and decisions. Institutions could only tolerate the refusal to cooperate for short periods and would soon resort to performance-management mechanisms against individual practitioners, who would probably be removed from their positions. They would thus contribute little to their cause, other than possibly generating some negative publicity. Total rejection of all instrumental values, then, is likely to be unrealistic and self-defeating.

To attempt an accommodation between the goods of effectiveness and the goods of excellence without losing sight of the latter requires a degree of compromise and may only be possible when the practice is in good order. The effectiveness demands and values of the institution do seem to affect the values of those nurses who move up the managerial ladder. As they are promoted, they often find that their capacity for independent action is more limited than they imagined when they were at the lower level. Thus the old conundrum that change can only occur from within a system, but that the system will change the individual before the individual reaches a position of sufficient influence to effect change, seems to hold true in the institutions of health care. Maintaining a practice in good order, then, requires a commitment to the core values of the practice. This requires staying true to the set of ideals that many aspiring nurses assume will be in abundance in nursing. In reality, the demands of nursing work make it difficult to sustain the ideal of service, or the pursuit of goods of excellence.

The attempt to retain nursing as a practice requires mounting a conscious and constant resistance to the corrupting influence of the institution. This may be possible if individuals have the support of others who understand nursing as a practice, but is probably unsustainable without it. Indeed, even with the support of a practice in good order, the constant battle required to maintain the kind of integrity for genuine and authentic nursing practice may be a significant factor in the reported increase in moral distress among nurses (see, for example, Corley 2002).

None of these options offers an easy answer to the challenge of maintaining the core values of nursing against the tide of instrumental values of the current, seemingly insatiable, managerialist appetite for more and more change forced upon practitioners under the political rhetoric of modernization. Perhaps, then, MacIntyre is right to be pessimistic about the long-term chances of survival of practices in the fragmented modern world. If nursing is to retain its core values, including those of care, compassion and trustworthiness, there is a real need for the institutions in which nursing takes place to work in ways that enable, rather than disable, individual nurses in pursuing the goods of practice-based excellence. Institutions, then, need to begin to act in ways that demonstrate due regard for the values of health and social care practices in general, and the practice of nursing in particular.

RESPONSE
Christine Hockley

In this response, I adopt a personal reflective approach, linking my work as a nurse in emergency care to the chapter contents. This response reflects my own reaction to and interpretation of the chapter; it does not necessarily represent the views of either the profession of adult nursing as a whole, or that of my colleagues working in emergency care.

As a nurse who trained in the early 1980s, I have had first-hand experience of the constant change in the way nursing is organized, delivered and monitored that is mentioned in the chapter. This has led many staff to test and question their own values, particularly in relation to the caring, compassionate, honest and trustworthy 'essence' of nursing practice, which both the nursing profession and the general public expect nurses to adhere to.

In many walks of life change is to be expected, and the health care professions are no exception. Great technological advances in both science and medicine have produced inevitable changes within these fields. Public demand for new treatments and services necessarily carry resource implications. This, coupled with the need for individual trusts to compete for the delivery of services, has led to many health care workers adopting a set of 'managerial' or 'instrumental values', emphasizing value for money, achievement of government set targets, and obtaining higher positions in the hospital league tables at whatever cost.

The field of emergency care is not excepted from change, targets and league tables (Department of Health 2004). Most nurses would allow that targets have been adopted in an attempt to improve patient care; the targets for emergency departments require that patients are seen, assessed, have any necessary diagnostic tests undertaken, and are safely discharged, transferred or admitted within four hours of their arrival at the department. This target has, for the majority of trusts, ended the previous state of affairs where patients were observed lying on trolleys for hours in corridors whilst waiting for a bed – a situation that was unacceptable, and had also caused many staff to question the values that were supposedly held by a 'caring' profession.

Despite this kind of situation being rare rather than the norm, our core values are still being tested. The need to achieve the four-hour target appears to have become all-consuming. Using large computer screens within the treatment areas, tracking systems identify patients who are in the department, continuously monitoring their length of stay with a coloured code which changes with each passing hour. When patients are discharged or admitted they are removed from the screens. Patients who are approaching the four-hour target time are then in danger of 'breaching' and the computer flashes warning signals. If the patient is not removed from the system before four hours is reached, their details turn red and they are officially referred to as having 'breached'. The nurse in charge then has to account to a senior manager for the reasons for non-compliance.

The public are aware of this type of system as it can now be seen in the hospital dramas and soap operas on television. Senior managers, amongst others, have access to the tracking system. They can therefore adopt the role of 'big brother', watching from a distance. While they may often claim that they are trying to help in the avoidance of a breach, the constant phone calls to remind nurses in charge tend to hinder, rather than help, the situation. This occurs at a time when a decision has to be made either to rapidly, and maybe unnecessarily, admit the patient, risk their unsafe discharge, or remove them from the tracking system, thereby denying their presence in the department and so allowing the 'instrumental' values to dominate and corrupt the institution and caring practice.

The numbers of breaches that a department experiences are closely monitored and penalties are incurred by trusts who fail to meet the targets. The current standard is that 98% of patients should be seen within four hours. Whilst the majority of patients will be seen within this time, there are also those who will, inevitably, breach. There are, of course, exceptions to the four-hour target; a patient who is seriously ill and needing intensive support to stabilize them before they are transferred out of the department serves as a good example of this.

Were the nurse in charge to be asked by managers or senior doctors in the department to stop the breach by requesting that they 'click the patient off as they will be going to the ward soon', in reality, the nurse would know that the porters were aware of this patient needing to be transferred but that they were busy elsewhere. The patient may still need to go for an X-ray before being admitted to the ward. By removing the patient from the computer screen the breach would, technically, have been avoided. This can be equated to MacIntyre's description of playing chess for external reward; the nurse would have played the game, the target would have been achieved, and no breach would have been recorded. But the nurse would have been dishonest and would not have adhered to nursing's intrinsic values.

If this were to happen, despite being removed from the computer screen, the patient would remain (at least temporarily) within the department and, therefore, still the responsibility of the nurse caring for them. The patient would now be in some 'virtual' area. They would not appear as a patient on a ward as they would not yet have arrived there, and they would no longer be shown on the emergency department screens. This would not absolve the nurse of the responsibility towards the patient and would violate nursing's values of caring, compassion, trustworthiness and honesty. All that would have occurred would be the adoption of 'instrumental values' to minimize the hassle the nurse would otherwise be subjected to. Fundamentally, this is dishonest.

The nature of emergency care is, by definition, unpredictable. The nurses working within it are used to pressure and the need for flexibility. Being pressurized to get patients out of the department and home before a safe discharge has been arranged, using accepted risk-management techniques, is not acceptable. Furthermore, admitting patients to inappropriate wards, as a 'transit stop' because the bed they have been properly allocated is not ready to accept them, causes concern to many nurses as they find their nursing values are threatened and that they are not adhering to the professional Code (NMC 2008).

One could then concur with MacIntyre when he argues that the aims of the institutions are fundamentally at odds with the aims of practice. He is not alone in thinking this. Thompson, Melia and Boyd (2000) argue that the business ethic of management may challenge the values of health care professionals. When discussing such issues with those in management positions, they claim to hold similar values to those identified by the nurses, even though this is not often evident in practice. They, too, have targets to meet and consequences to face if these are not achieved. Whilst one can accept that the management of health care does, and always will, require some bureaucracy, the administration of that bureaucracy must be honest and transparent if the values expected of all health care professionals are to be upheld.

What is needed is equilibrium between what MacIntyre calls internal and external goods (or goods of excellence and goods of effectiveness respectively). Personally, I have observed how such a balance can work. The senior nurses within my department have all agreed, and have informed the managers and medical staff, that we will do all that is possible to avoid any patient breaches and strive to achieve the required targets. We will not, however, 'fudge the figures to achieve a target'. This honest approach has had numerous benefits because it has revealed previously unseen obstacles that may have prevented us achieving the target. In many cases, the system has been altered or improved and all of this has resulted in a benefit to patient care.

I recently asked a group of second-year student nurses to identify what they believed were the core values that both they, and the general public, expected nurses to adhere to. Despite nursing and the role of the nurse being very different in the twenty-first century, the core values of caring, beneficence, non-malificence, compassion, honesty and justice remain the same as they were in the days of Florence Nightingale. It is not the values that have changed, but the context, and the manner, in which they are interpreted and tested.

REFERENCES

Corley, M.C. (2002) 'Nurse moral distress: a proposed theory and research agenda.' *Nursing Ethics 9*, 6, 636–650.

Department of Health (2004) *Reforming Emergency Care.* London: Department of Health.

Flemming, K. and Fenton, M. (2002) 'Making Sense of Research Evidence to Inform Decision Making.' In C. Thompson and D. Dowding (eds) *Clinical Decision Making and Judgement in Nursing.* Edinburgh: Churchill Livingstone, pp.109–129.

Gerth, H.H. and Mills, C.W. (eds) (1948) *From Max Weber: Essays in Sociology.* London: Routledge and Kegan Paul.

Handy, C. (1996) *Beyond Certainty.* London: Arrow Books.

Lassman, P. (2000) 'The Rule of Man over Man: Politics, Power and Legitimation.' In S. Turner (ed.) *The Cambridge Companion to Weber.* Cambridge: Cambridge University Press, pp.83–98.

Lewin, K. (1951) *Field Theory in Social Sciences.* New York: Harper and Row.

MacIntyre, A. (1985) *After Virtue: A Study in Moral Theory* (2nd edn). London: Duckworth.

MacIntyre, A. (1988) *Whose Justice? Which Rationality?* London: Duckworth.

Nursing and Midwifery Council (NMC) (2008) *The Code: Standards of Conduct, Performance and Ethics for Nurses and Midwives.* London: NMC.

Paley, J. (2006) 'Evidence and expertise.' *Nursing Inquiry 13*, 2, 82–93.

Pattison, S. (1997) *The Faith of the Managers: When Management Becomes Religion.* London: Cassell.

Power, M. (1997) *The Audit Society: Rituals of Verification.* Oxford: Oxford University Press.

Rolfe, G., Segrott, J. and Jordan, S. (2008) 'Tensions and contradictions in nurses' perceptions of evidence-based practice.' *Journal of Nursing Management 16*, 4, 440–451.

Scottish Intercollegiate Guidelines Network (SIGN) (2002) *A Guide to Developer's Handbook.* Edinburgh: SIGN.

Sockett, H. (1993) *The Moral Base for Teacher Professionalism.* New York: Teachers College Press.

Sellman, D. (1997) 'The virtues in the moral education of nurses: Florence Nightingale revisited.' *Nursing Ethics 4*, 1, 3–11.

Sellman, D. (2000) 'Alasdair MacIntyre and the practice of nursing.' *Nursing Philosophy 1*, 1, 26–33.

Thompson, I., Melia, K. and Boyd, K. (2000) *Nursing Ethics* (4th edn). London: Churchill Livingstone.

Chapter 7

The Profession of Pharmacy in the United Kingdom: Changing Values?

David Badcott

INTRODUCTION

The practice of pharmacy has a long history. Yet it was not until 1841 with the foundation of the Pharmaceutical Society of Great Britain, later the Royal Pharmaceutical Society of Great Britain (RPSGB), that pharmacy became established as an independent profession in this country. Prior to that, many of the activities subsequently associated with pharmacy had been undertaken by apothecaries (who were both physicians and compounders of medicines), and by druggists or grocers who dealt directly with members of the public in various bulk drugs.

During the past 40 or 50 years, the nature of retail (community) pharmacy and hospital pharmacy has changed markedly. Extemporaneous compounding of medicines in the pharmacy has been replaced by dispensing of industrially manufactured proprietary alternatives, and dispensing is now mostly as standard patient pre-packs containing patient information leaflets. Computer-printed labels have replaced handwritten labels, and automatic database checks on dosage and therapeutic incompatibilities are routine. Prescriptions are written in the English language rather than medical Latin. Because many traditional professional duties have been superseded, pharmacists can now devote much more time to an active patient-centred role, progressively undertaking additional treatment responsibilities and promoting health by providing advice on matters such as smoking reduction, heart disease, diabetes, stroke, cancer, under-18 contraception, obesity in children, long-term illnesses, substance misuse and immunization.

Most health care professions, including pharmacy, have codes of practice or of ethics that frame their ethos and are intended to guide the behaviour of their membership. This chapter examines the relevance and nature of the Pharmaceutical Society's Code of Ethics to the changing nature of pharmacy and the extent to which the Code reflects appropriate moral, professional or other values.

THE NATURE OF PHARMACY PRACTICE

Pharmacists have provided valuable services particularly to local communities over very many generations. These include dispensing of doctors' prescriptions, and providing associated therapeutic guidance for patients. Since the advent of the National Health Service (NHS) in 1948 the vast majority of prescriptions are NHS, with the patient paying a standard fee per item unless otherwise exempted (although NHS prescription charges were abolished entirely in Wales from April 2007, and are expected to end in Northern Ireland in April 2010 and in Scotland in 2011). Pharmacists also give advice on common medical ailments, and sell over-the-counter (OTC) medicines along with multiple non-medical products and services such as cosmetics and toiletries.

As well as 'community pharmacies', pharmacy departments in stores such as Boots the Chemists are commonplace, as are the growing numbers of supermarkets with integral pharmacies. In these premises, the pharmacy might be seen as just another retail outlet like those found in the busy high street. It is almost certainly because of the somewhat hybrid nature of community or retail pharmacy – being both a commercial business operation with competitive retail selling as a major component and a provider of professional health-related services – that the status of pharmacy as a profession has sometimes been disputed. There is, perhaps, a suspicion that community pharmacy cannot be a 'proper profession' because it engages in retail trade by selling things and making a profit (Caldwell 2007).

So what really does characterize a profession? A basic general view might be that a profession is simply an occupational body whose members have followed, and been examined on, a prescribed course of training, with ongoing membership then conditional on the espousal of that society's declared values and objectives (particularly in relationships with the general public). Barber (1988) favours a definition of professional behaviour in terms of four essential attributes. These are:

- possession of a body of generalized, systematic knowledge

- a concern with the interests of the community, as opposed to self-interest

- the existence of ethical codes to guide behaviour (and which are transmitted through processes of socialization)

- reward systems that recognize work achievement, rather than promoting self-interest.

The eligibility of pharmacy as a profession is reviewed by Harding and Taylor (1997). The authors express concern that the move to undertake broader duties in public health may undermine the primary claim of professional status as medicinal drug experts. There seems little doubt that pharmacy is a profession when characterized in general terms and more specifically by those activities directly related to health care (see further: Bissell and Traulsen 2005). Health care practice is arguably among the areas of employment in which espousing moral values is essential – and having both commercial objectives and espousing those caring values most often associated with health care professions need not be mutually incompatible. All health care professionals expect to receive a monetary reward (salary or professional fee) for their services and so are, in that sense, commercial. And having professional status extends beyond the daytime job. Pharmacists, together with other groups of health care professionals, are expected to conduct themselves both on and off duty in a way that does not bring the profession into disrepute. MacIntyre (1999) supports the notion that individuals should not adopt different role-based moral postures (such as in private life and in professional life):

> To have integrity is to refuse to be, to have educated oneself so that one is no longer able to be, one kind of person in one social context, while quite another in other contexts. It is to have set inflexible limits to one's adaptability to the roles that one may be called upon to play. (p.317)

Levy (1976) whilst acknowledging that 'To be a professional practitioner is to give up some of one's autonomy and to relinquish some of one's rights as a freely functioning human being' (p.113), nevertheless emphasizes the possible problems of conflicts both within personal values and between personal and professional values. But for pharmacy, there is a need to ensure that having inflexible limits means not only maintaining appropriate conduct in private life but also not allowing commercial criteria to take precedence over, or to compromise, care-related considerations. The array of espoused values of a profession must be consistent and non-contradictory. Thus those who practise a profession like pharmacy with both commercial and health care-related aims cannot have a mission statement of 'maximizing profits' without ensuring that commercial aims should never be prioritized over ethical obligations. (See Resnik, Ranelli and Resnik 2000 for a discussion of some possible conflicts between ethics and business in community pharmacy.)

A TIME OF CONTINUING CHANGE IN PHARMACY

Major changes have occurred in the technical aspects of community pharmacy practice during recent decades. The term 'deskilling' has been applied to describe the effect of these changes. The now largely defunct activities such as extemporaneous preparation of medicines (for example 'mixtures' or ointments) are basically craft skills essentially relying on practical training and the application of experience. Nevertheless, at the same time, pharmacy has undergone marked changes both in educational standards (by extending the period of formal academic training by an additional year, from three years to four), and also in the composition of the academic curriculum. New graduates now are more comprehensively qualified in terms of their knowledge of the actions and applications of medicinal drugs in therapeutics. They also have appropriate practical training in pharmacy practice, and with the inclusion of social pharmacy and pharmacy ethics in the curriculum are more able to deliver improving standards of care to patients. Fortuitously, therefore, technical changes have been accompanied by equally profound changes in opportunities for the profession to adopt both a more caring and intellectually rigorous stance in its practice.

The opportunities for pharmacists to undertake a wider role in community health have been recognized by successive governments and others. A Nuffield Committee report on Pharmacy (Nuffield Foundation 1986) concluded that the application of pharmacists' knowledge and skills could be extended to assist better general practice prescribing and to advise patients on using their medication. UK government appointee Sir Derek Wanless produced two influential reports relevant to pharmacy centred on potential initiatives in health care: *Securing Our Future Health – Taking a Long-term View* (Wanless 2002; see also Royal Pharmaceutical Society of Great Britain 2003), and *Securing Good Health for the Whole Population* (Wanless 2004). Within these Wanless proposals pharmacy is perceived as a major untapped resource, with considerable potential in the fields of chronic disease management, prescribing advice and treatment optimization, and what might be termed public health initiatives.

The relevant sequel to these reports for pharmacy is a document titled *Choosing Health through Pharmacy. A Programme for Pharmaceutical Public Health 2005–2015* (Department of Health 2005). This 85-page strategy document lists 22 key features including:

- The public health challenge, the importance of building on the strengths of pharmacy, the evidence base for pharmaceutical public health and the contribution that pharmacy can make in different sectors.

- The key role of pharmacists and their staff in providing information and advice to the public on health improvement, and in providing signposting to other services.

- How pharmacists and their staff can identify individuals with risk factors for disease offering them lifestyle assessments.

- The contribution of pharmacy to the care of people with long-term conditions, e.g. heart disease, diabetes and asthma, by encouraging the effective use of medicines; promoting healthy lifestyles; supporting self-care; carrying out medication reviews; managing disease systematically within multi-professional teams; and working in partnership with case managers.

(Department of Health 2005, pp.7–8)

The changes in pharmacy practice can be summarized as:

- transformation of many key aspects of the traditional prescription-dispensing service

- recognition of the role of patient care as being central to the whole ethos, not only of pharmacy practice but also of all branches of health care and medicine

- a revised and extended role for pharmacists in patient-oriented medicines management and aspects of public health

- opportunities for pharmacists to 'counter prescribe' from an increasing list of some of the more potent medicines rescheduled from prescription only (POM) classification to pharmacy (P)

- supplementary prescribing by appropriately trained pharmacists to prescribe any medicine (including controlled drugs) within the framework of a patient-specific clinical management plan approved by a medical doctor.

The drivers for change within pharmacy are therefore due partly to initiatives from within the profession, prompted and enabled by political pressures and initiatives from central government – particularly with regard to plans for major overhaul of the NHS and for better provision of public health. Acknowledgement of the centrality of patient care in pharmacy is perhaps fortuitous for the profession, since it fits well with many of the more patient-centred changes envisaged above. The fact that a parliamentary All-Party Pharmacy Group was founded in 1999 with the aim of raising awareness of the profession of pharmacy and promoting the contribution of pharmacists to the health of the nation is perhaps a formal recognition of the potential for pharmacists to play a fuller part in a more personalized health care.

CHANGING PHARMACY VALUES?

With these substantial practice changes in mind, a key question is: will the values that underpinned community pharmacy in the past still be appropriate? To address this question, it is first advantageous to consider the conceptual nature of the relationship between patient and pharmacist, and to ask whether that relationship still holds or whether it needs amendment. I shall propose that the pharmaceutical care provided by pharmacists for patients in dispensing prescriptions, counselling on safe and effective treatment, encouraging medicines-use reviews and providing advice on broader issues of public health tacitly recognizes a context of vulnerability, obligation, trust, and respect for patient autonomy. These are contextual moral considerations that generally situate the relationship between patient and health care practitioner. They therefore seem to fit all categories of the latter (e.g. medical doctors, nurses, pharmacists, osteopaths, etc.) in virtually all circumstances.

Patients are vulnerable in a number of important respects. First, they are vulnerable to the disease for which they are seeking treatment. This state of vulnerability provokes them, or prompts a relative or carer, to seek advice or treatment from someone (a medical doctor or other health care provider) who they believe to be qualified and knowledgeable, and who can properly diagnose and treat their condition. Second, they (patients) are at least potentially (and sometimes actually) vulnerable to the treatments they receive. Treatments need to be both safe and effective. Adverse drug reactions are far more common than we might like to believe (serious, so-called 'side-effects' may not be detected until large numbers of patients have received a medication) and proof-of-efficacy studies cannot deliver absolute therapeutic certainty. This theoretical and practical knowledge of therapeutic and prophylactic medicines continues to be a crucial component of pharmaceutical expertise. Indeed, Harding and Taylor (1997, p.547) assert that 'pharmacy has the necessary knowledge base to control the symbolic transformation of the pharmacological entity – the drug – into the social object – the medicine, yet has failed to capitalise on this when attempting to define its professional role'.

It is because of the state of vulnerability of the (potential) patient, and because the health care practitioner undertakes to help, that a professional obligation is incurred. We assume that obligation is a fundamental aspect of being a professional in any walk of life, but particularly in health care: '…your special responsibilities (as a pharmacist or other health care professional) derive from the fact other people are dependent upon you and are particularly vulnerable to your actions and choices' (Goodin 1985, p.33). Being a pharmacist, or being a nurse, automatically brings about just that state and sense of dependent obligation. A sense of obligation is the value that links all health care professionals with patients for whom they care. It is common and fundamental values that also connect health care professionals with each other. Furthermore, the recognition of vulnerability and obligation can only flourish in an atmosphere of complete trust. Trust is paramount. Why should you follow my advice if you don't trust me, particularly if your life may be at stake?

A further significant moral concept in health care relationships is autonomy: permitting/encouraging a competent person to make their own decisions concerning their wellbeing and future. This applies equally to patients or clients as to health care practitioner colleagues. I am attracted to the term and concept of 'principled autonomy' adopted by Stirrat and Gill (2005) with acknowledgement of O'Neill's (2002) work on 'trust'. Principled autonomy captures the notion that patients should always have a major say in their treatment subject to competence. And here I mean 'competence' both in the specific sense of being mentally able (in other words, not being mentally impaired), but also reflecting the more general meaning of being 'knowledgeably' capable. Thus receipt of advice on personal medication or perhaps on lifestyle-related issues such as smoking, excessive alcohol consumption or obesity will hinge on the patient or customer's preparedness to listen and an ability to understand and apply – even though the context is one of volition. A key difference perhaps is that a pharmacist's advice on prescribed medicines has more implied force than in the area of public health (where pharmacists have a need to establish public confidence and perhaps that of other health care professionals), though related issues of compliance, adherence and concordance would appear to be much the same.

So, just which moral or other values are most appropriate for pharmacy practice as it continues to evolve at the present time? The 'vulnerability; obligation; trust; autonomy' conceptual model as described would have been appropriate for pharmacy in previous decades even though the importance of patient care was neither formally stated nor recognized. The sort of moral values indicated by More (2003) as standards for judging conduct (honesty, fairness, altruism, kindness, justice) form a useful basic nucleus of values for pharmacy, though it is appropriate to append those of beneficence, non-maleficence, and respect for personal dignity and autonomy, which are becoming well-recognized in modern health care practice generally (see, for example, Beauchamp and Childress 2008). Importantly, these are all values that accord well with the vulnerability model.

The enhancement of pharmaceutical services into more obvious personal patient care, public health promotion and into providing other therapeutic advice would be unlikely to benefit from substantially expanding the *content* of a list of values relevant to general pharmacy practice: there are at present no obvious omissions. What *should* change, and is changing, is the necessity of emphasizing the vital importance of values and the development of an increased awareness of the role of values and ethical principles in professional pharmacy care.

THE RPSGB CODE OF ETHICS

Although the RPSGB was founded in 1841, a formal code of ethics (which was really a code of business practice) did not come into use until 1939 and then largely focused on prohibiting unacceptable trade practices, with very little attention given to moral issues in respect of patients or customers. As Rodgers and John (2006) indicate:

> The first code of ethics was to form the basis against which cases of unprofessional conduct would be measured by the Statutory Committee. In keeping with the times, the statement was paternalistic with the Society concentrating on setting out a list of activities in which the pharmacist was not allowed to participate. Predominant among these was a prohibition on advertising with five of the eleven statements banning various forms of advertisement. Inducements such as gifts or price-cutting were disallowed. Of the basic ethical principles only non-maleficence is evident. This is seen in the requirements not to discuss medication with a patient in a way that might impair confidence in the prescriber and not to sell medicines suspected of being obtained for purposes of abuse. (p.722)

With the exception of maintaining patient and prescriber confidence and curbing substance abuse, the Code can be seen as a code of practice reflecting business solidarity and a desire to maintain the reputation of the profession. It is essentially business-centred and provides little that could be thought of as ethical consideration for the patient. Instead, the Code reflects broadly those utilitarian *economic values* used to judge goods and services (More 2003) that were deemed to be appropriate for pharmacy in the immediate pre-World War II period and earlier.

To all intents and purposes, the practice of pharmacy in the UK is monopolistic. With the exception of certain non-prescription and generally less potent medicines that are on the General Sales List (and therefore available for sale in supermarkets and other trade outlets), and 'dispensing doctors', only registered practising pharmacists are legally and exclusively authorized to undertake certain duties concerning the handling and sale of listed poisons and medicines, and dispensing of medical prescriptions. Pharmacists must be registered with the RPSGB, the statutory body that currently controls pharmacists, pharmaceutical premises and the practice of pharmacy. In view of the strict legal regulation of poisons and medicines, the RPSGB Code of Ethics was, until recently, predominantly a guide to handling these. The system of regulatory inspection operated by the RPSGB is informed both by relevant legislation and an understanding by members that the Code is mandatory. A legally constituted statutory committee adjudicates possible breaches. Changes are currently in hand to create two separate bodies to, first, exercise statutory regulation (a General Pharmaceutical Council is expected to be in place by January 2010), and to, second, establish a newly constituted professional association.

From 1999 onwards, there has been a clearly recognizable move towards a code of practice with a substantial focus on ethical considerations. A consultation document in that year ('Pharmacists' ethics and professional performance') sought members' views on a draft proposal 'to set a framework in the new millennium' that included not only 'bread and butter' service performance specifications, but brief statements on 'pharmacists' ethics' and 'The role and accountability of a pharmacist' (Royal Pharmaceutical Society of Great Britain 1999). Part I (Pharmacists' Ethics) included several statements or themes that emphasize a growing awareness by the RPSGB of the need for pharmacists to engage with the basics of an ethical understanding of their role in health care. These included: the need for pharmacists to engage with ethics as the study of moral choices, and the importance of the values underpinning these; and the place of ethics in balancing competing rights and responsibilities, and the fluidity of ethical principles and their sensitivity to wider environments.

Further contribution to a debate on a revised code of ethics was provided with publication of a report from the RPSGB's Core Values Working Party: *Developing Pharmacy Values: Stimulating the Debate* (Cribb and Barber 2000). This paper strongly argues the benefit of encouraging pharmacists to become more versed in ('literate about, and engaged with') value issues, and advocates further debate and consultation on some of the major issues, with the institution of appropriate teaching on values and society, and the fostering of interdisciplinary research in pharmacy, the humanities and social sciences. Whilst there is useful discussion of the sort of values that might frame a revitalized pharmacy code, such as the four-component mantra of Beauchamp and Childress (2008) – beneficence, non-maleficence, autonomy and justice – as well as general professional, vocational and institutional values, there is reluctance to deliver or prescribe a definitive list of core pharmacy values. Nevertheless, the authors recognize the importance of identifying values that would emphasize the nature and application of the technical expertise of pharmacists as medicines authorities, and which might also resonate with a growing public realization of the importance of pharmaceutical care.

An article written by the chairman of the RPSGB council's ethics working party prefaced publication of a revised code (Darling 2001):

> The revised code, in line with trends in government health care policy, puts patients at the centre for care... The three-tier approach of Principles, Obligations and Guidance supplemented by Standards of Good Professional Practice has gone. In its place we have developed a code that identifies pharmacists' key professional responsibilities of beneficence, competence and integrity, and encourages pharmacists to consider these responsibilities when deciding how to resolve the dilemmas faced in everyday practice... The rulebook approach of earlier codes of ethics has been replaced by a document which empowers pharmacists to develop their own practice in accordance with the key responsibilities. (p.589)

Importantly, the 2001 Code incorporated a new 'conscience clause' in which provision is made for pharmacists having conscientious objections (relating to religious belief, personal conviction or inadequate training) to decline from providing certain services, subject to having informed and agreed with their employer and being prepared to advise a patient or customer where that service could be obtained.

Consultations on a further revision of the Code of Ethics that would apply both to pharmacists and pharmacy technicians were undertaken in June 2006 (Council of the Royal Pharmaceutical Society of Great Britain 2006a) and November 2006 (Council of the Royal

Pharmaceutical Society of Great Britain 2006b). A key change indicated in these consultations was that a revised code would be based on 'seven (mandatory) principles of ethical pharmacy practice (that express the values central to the identity of the pharmacy professions)'. The seven principles, together with explanatory paragraphs are intended to '…inform the conduct, performance and practice of registered pharmacy professionals':

- Make the care of the patient your first concern.

- Exercise your professional judgement in the interests of patients and the public.

- Show respect for others.

- Encourage patients to participate in decisions about their care.

- Develop your professional knowledge and competence.

- Be honest and trustworthy.

- Take responsibility for your working practices.

The new Code incorporating the seven principles came into force on 1 August 2007. The earlier 'conscience clause' remains in place under the heading 'Show respect for others': 'Ensure that if your religious or moral beliefs prevent you from providing a particular professional service, the relevant persons or authorities are informed of this and patients are referred to alternative providers for the service they require' (Royal Pharmaceutical Society of Great Britain 2007, p.8).

Some months prior to publication of the current Code (Royal Pharmaceutical Society of Great Britain 2007), a report urging the reorientation of core pharmacy values was introduced (Benson, Cribb and Barber 2007). The report followed an empirical research study undertaken 'To explore and map the values and ethics of pharmacy practitioners (mainly, but not exclusively from conventional, that is, community practice) through their self-reported day-to-day perceptions and experiences' (p.3). The authors acknowledged that their findings were not statistically representative but claimed that the recorded narratives provide useful illustrations of some of the ethical and other values *theoretically generalizable* to pharmacy practice. The summary report makes available a useful analysis of the major influences on the changing status and nature of pharmacy practice:

- Growth in clinical roles.

- Nature of accountability becoming more complex.

- Membership of a multi-disciplinary team and shared care.

- Increasing patient expectations for involvement in own care.

- Cultural and religious diversity.

- Wider responsibilities to society for equitable, efficient and economic use of resources.

(Benson *et al.* 2007, pp.22–23)

The report correctly identifies as 'obvious needs' that greater attention be paid to the ethical concepts of, first, patient autonomy and distributive justice and, second, quality or value of life, and makes recommendations that include the need to improve the day-to-day identification and management of dilemmas and decisions.

CONCLUSIONS

So, what are we to make of the new principle-based RPSGB 2007 Code? I am assuming that (moral) values and moral principles are inextricably linked and to some extent at least may be thought of as different facets of the same notion. Generally, we take it that moral principles are basic, fundamental, law-like or deontological statements, such as 'Do not kill'. The 'principles' of the RPSGB Code of Ethics are foundational policy statements that seek to emphasize and clarify the obligations of those engaged in the profession and practice of pharmacy. As stated, the seven principles and their supporting explanations encapsulate what it means to be a registered pharmacist or pharmacy technician. A series of professional standards and guidance documents that expand on the principles and some of the key aspects, such as patient consent and confidentiality, support the Code.

It is not difficult to identify within the Code commonly expressed moral values such as respect (for the person, their interests, their privacy and their autonomy, irrespective of cultural or other difference), honesty, trust, integrity and confidentiality. The possibility of competing interests reflecting the commercial/health care duality of pharmacy is dealt with in section 2.1: 'Make sure that your professional judgment is not impaired by personal or commercial interests, incentives, targets and similar measures'. (This in the context of acting only in the best interests of individual patients and the public.)

All in all, the Code is a considerable advance over previous, less 'values-minded' editions and sets the right tone in a much more caring-conscious era of health care. Strictly speaking, the code is actually a code of practice with an ethical flavour and not really a code of ethics. Furthermore, because it is mandatory, there is perhaps a danger of observing the Code simply because to do otherwise could result in sanction – get caught breaking the Code and you are punished. In other words, there is little to distinguish the Code and a formal legal requirement. Such being the case, the Code's authors perhaps misunderstand the crucial difference that we (should) behave ethically because we believe that it is the right thing to do and not because we fear being punished. But to some extent this perhaps reflects the necessarily highly regulated environment of dealing with potent medicines which in the extreme can influence life or death. Wittgenstein (2001) neatly encapsulates the fitting teleological nature of moral behaviour:

> It is clear, however, that ethics is nothing to do with punishment and reward in the normal sense of these words …
> There must indeed be some kind of ethical reward and ethical punishment, but they must reside in the action itself. (p.86)

The thrust of modern health care ethics, particularly of virtue ethics or ethics of care, is on the rightness of an action for its own sake, and there is a risk that this aspect may be largely eclipsed by the tone of professional codes of ethics such as that of the RPSGB (you must; your conduct will be judged). And there is perhaps a further debatable point as to the relationship between personal values ('one's principles or standards, one's judgment of what is valuable or important in life, such as honesty, fairness, altruism, kindness, justice'), and, for example, corporate or professional values, which generally intend to set out that body's generalized values stance for the benefit of the public and to provide standards for judging conduct. Perhaps pharmacists, in becoming increasingly more of a caring profession, should be encouraged toward embracing the principles of virtue ethics as generally favoured in nursing, rather than being threatened with a big stick. After all, 'The principles' rightly direct attention first and foremost toward the patient: make the care of patients your first concern. In so doing, pharmacists would themselves gradually develop an appropriate set of moral values. The report of Benson *et al.* (2007) correctly highlights the need for greater familiarity with ethical concepts and to improve 'identification and management of ethical and value components within day-to-day practice dilemmas and decisions'. The new Code and an increasing awareness of the importance of moral values in pharmacy professional practice will contribute to developing an atmosphere in which ethical behaviour is considered to be as important and commonplace as technical competence.

RESPONSE
Alan Nathan

I agree with David Badcott's assessment that pharmacy is undergoing fundamental change. The need for pharmacists' manipulative and small-scale formulation skills to prepare medicines extemporaneously in the pharmacy has gone. It is being replaced by the enhanced clinical skills required to advise patients and other health professionals on the use and selection of modern medicines, which are much more effective than their predecessors but also potentially much more harmful if prescribed or used incorrectly. However, community pharmacists still operate in a largely commercial environment, and this can present barriers to community pharmacists being able to practise fully in accordance with health care values and the principles of the RPSGB Code of Ethics. (Hospital pharmacists, on the other hand, who account for about 20% of practising pharmacists, are fully integrated members of health care teams in a non-commercial environment and are able much more easily to espouse and practise in accordance with ethical values). The law relating to medicines in the UK can also create barriers to ethical pharmaceutical practice.

Despite the transition toward a more clinically orientated role, the financial viability of community pharmacy still depends largely on the supply of merchandise. Even though more than 90 per cent of that is medicines dispensed against NHS prescriptions, it is remunerated largely on a 'per item supplied' basis, and the emerging clinical services are also mainly paid for on a piecework basis. This is in contrast to the way most other NHS health professionals are rewarded, either as salaried employees or, in the case of general practitioners, on a per patient basis for the provision of holistic health care. Other primary health care providers, such as dentists, are also paid partly on an item of service basis, and general practitioners' remuneration is enhanced through achieving performance targets, such as for immunizations and various types of health screening. Although some of these practitioners, as well as health professionals practising privately, may be tempted to increase their income by providing unnecessary treatments or services, they are independent practitioners and have only to answer to their own consciences.

The situation for many community pharmacists is different. Community pharmacies are increasingly owned by large multiples. These are public limited companies, or in the case of the largest, a private equity company. The majority of community pharmacists are now employees working for these companies, which operate in a commercial environment where competition is intense and the traditional over-the-counter, non-medicinal trade and even medicines sales are being lost to supermarkets and internet traders. There is therefore great pressure from management on pharmacists in their branches to maximize profit from NHS pharmaceutical services. This is being achieved in some cases through staff reductions, putting pressure on pharmacists to operate under conditions that they may feel are unsafe and contravene the profession's Code of Ethics, and which may undermine the principle of non-maleficence. But they tend to accept such conditions as they fear being disciplined by their employers or losing their jobs if they complain.

A new NHS contract for community pharmacy was introduced in 2005, under which the profits on the purchase and supply of medicines were substantially reduced, with the intention of using some of the money saved to finance new clinical services. One of the services that has been instituted is medicines use review (MUR), which is paid for on a per review basis – with a pharmacy allowed to carry out up to 400 per year. Patients are supposed to be selected for review on the basis of clinical need by pharmacists using their professional judgement, and a review is supposed to take around half an hour altogether. There are reliable reports that some multiple pharmacy companies are coercing pharmacists to perform the full quota of reviews, regardless of real need and as quickly and perfunctorily as possible. Pharmacists are also usually required to carry out reviews without any extra staffing. This situation could compromise a pharmacist's integrity.

Pharmacists' practice is closely controlled by the Medicines Act 1968, the law governing the supply of medicines. This is now over 40 years old and the direct descendant of a line of legislation going back more than a century. It is formulated to regulate medicines supply from pharmacies essentially by traders rather than health professionals, as pharmacies can be, and many are, owned by non-pharmacists (by now the majority, as independent pharmacy owners retire and sell their businesses to multiples). As a result, the Medicines Act is very restrictive and severe – even the most minor dispensing error is a criminal offence – and pharmacists work with this at the back of their minds. Their overriding instinct is, therefore, to practise defensively to avoid any risk of breaking the law, which can undermine the principle of beneficence. For example, pharmacists will often refuse to use the regulations in the Act which allow for supply of small quantities of previously prescribed medicines in an emergency without a prescription.

The situation has in fact been exacerbated in the past few years by the RPSGB. In a vain attempt to avoid losing its role as the profession's regulator it became much more rigorous in its pursuit of pharmacists for even the most minor professional breaches or misdemeanours, and this has further increased the trend to defensive practice.

The RPSGB could deal more effectively with the multiples and their superintendent pharmacists who are ultimately accountable for their companies' professional activities. Perhaps the new regulator (the General Pharmaceutical Council, which takes over in 2010) will take a more forceful approach to dealing with the multiples than the RPSGB appeared to. The Medicines Act could be amended so that minor dispensing errors are no longer treated as criminal offences, although there is no indication that this is likely to happen.

REFERENCES

Barber, B. (1988) 'Professions and Emerging Professions.' In J.C. Callahan (ed.) *Ethical Issues in Professional Life*. New York and Oxford: Oxford University Press.

Beauchamp, T. and Childress, J. (2008) *Principles of Biomedical Ethics* (6th edn). Oxford: Oxford University Press.

Benson, A., Cribb, A. and Barber, N. (2007) *Respect for Medicines and Respect for People: Mapping Pharmacist Practitioners' Perceptions and Experiences of Ethics and Values*. London: Royal Pharmaceutical Society of Great Britain.

Bissell, P. and Traulsen, J.M. (2005) *Sociology and Pharmacy Practice*. London: Pharmaceutical Press.

Caldwell, I. (2007) 'What does it mean to be a member of a profession in 21st century Britain?' *The Pharmaceutical Journal 278*, 7448, 461–462.

Council of the Royal Pharmaceutical Society of Great Britain (2006a) 'Consultation on a code of ethics: structure.' *Pharmaceutical Journal 276*, 727.

Council of the Royal Pharmaceutical Society of Great Britain (2006b) 'Consultation on a code of ethics: detailed content and wording.' *Pharmaceutical Journal 277*, 589.

Cribb, A. and Barber, N. (2000) *Developing Pharmacy Values: Stimulating the Debate.* London: Royal Pharmaceutical Society of Great Britain.

Darling, B. (2001) 'A new code of ethics and standards.' *Pharmaceutical Journal 266*, 589–596.

Department of Health (2005) *Choosing Health through Pharmacy. A Programme for Pharmaceutical Public Health 2005–2015.* London: Department of Health.

Goodin, R.E. (1985) *Protecting the Vulnerable.* Chicago, IL and London: University of Chicago Press.

Harding, G. and Taylor, K. (1997) 'Responding to change: the case of community pharmacy in Great Britain.' *Sociology of Health and Illness 19*, 5, 547–560.

Levy, C.S. (1976) 'Personal versus professional values: the practitioner's dilemmas.' *Clinical Social Work 4*, 2, 110–120.

MacIntyre, A. (1999) 'Social structures and their threats to moral agency.' *Philosophy 74*, 3, 311–329.

More, T.A. (2003) *Facts, Values and Decision-making in Recreational Resource Management.* Available at www.georgewright.org/0332more.pdf, accessed on 3 March 2007.

Nuffield Foundation (1986) *Nuffield Committee of Inquiry into Pharmacy.* London: The Nuffield Foundation.

O'Neill, O. (2002) *Autonomy and Trust in Bioethics.* Cambridge: Cambridge University Press.

Resnik, D., Ranelli, P. and Resnik, D. (2000) 'The conflict between ethics and business in community pharmacy: what about patient counselling?' *Journal of Business Ethics 28*, 2, 179–186.

Rodgers, R. and John, D. (2006) 'Paternalism to professional judgement – the history of the code of ethics.' *Pharmaceutical Journal 276*, 7405, 721–722.

Royal Pharmaceutical Society of Great Britain (1999) 'Pharmacists' ethics and professional performance. A consultation document on a new code of ethics.' *Pharmaceutical Journal 263*, CE1–CE10.

Royal Pharmaceutical Society of Great Britain (2003) *Securing Good Health for the Whole Population: The 'Wanless 2' Review.* Available at www.rpsgb.org.uk/pdfs/wanless2sub03.pdf, accessed on 20 July 2007.

Royal Pharmaceutical Society of Great Britain (2007) *Code of Ethics for Pharmacists and Pharmacy Technicians.* London: Royal Pharmaceutical Society of Great Britain.

Stirrat, G.M. and Gill, R. (2005) 'Autonomy in medical ethics after O'Neill.' *Journal of Medical Ethics 31*, 3, 127–130.

Wanless, D. (2002) *Securing Our Future Health: Taking a Long-term View.* London: HM Treasury.

Wanless, D. (2004) *Securing Good Health for the Whole Population.* London: HM Treasury.

Wittgenstein, L. (2001) *Tractatus Logico-Philosophicus* (Routledge *Classics*, 2nd edn, pbk). London: Routledge and Kegan Paul.

Chapter 8

Professional Values in Interaction: Non-directiveness, Client-centredness and Other-orientation in Genetic Counselling

Srikant Sarangi

INTRODUCTION

Can professional neutrality and client-centredness be reconciled with professional authority/knowledge and client autonomy/agency in situated encounters between professionals and clients? This chapter considers how dominant professional values in the context of genetic counselling may be incommensurable. Specifically, it examines two sets of professional values – client-centredness and non-directiveness – by undertaking a discourse analysis of real-life genetic counselling encounters. Given the familial basis of genetic conditions, both counsellors and clients routinely have to balance individual autonomy with an orientation to 'family–others'. This other-orientation plays a mediating role when discussions centre around decisions about genetic testing and disclosure of test results. Within the genetic counselling profession, the tension between being non-directive and being client-centred is acknowledged, and it provides the motivation for examining closely what transpires interactionally in counselling sessions.

THE RHETORIC OF 'PROFESSIONAL CORRECTNESS'

All professions have an altruistic orientation to clients-as-others, although this may mask their economic self-interests (Illich 1977). Genetic counselling, as an other-oriented professional activity, is understood as a communication and educational process to facilitate clients' understanding of the nature of genetic disorder and attendant decision-making processes. Historically, genetic counselling as a professional activity shares characteristics with other counselling and therapeutic activities such as psychotherapy but also with traditional medical consultation; this hybridity is routinely manifest at the interactional level (Sarangi 2000). Kessler (1979) identifies a shift from 'content-oriented counselling' (with a medical information focus) to a 'person-oriented counselling' (where clients are offered the opportunity to reflect on their situation from a psychological perspective). This connects with Rogers' (1951) call for 'client-centred therapy'.

Unlike in many counselling/therapeutic settings, the client-centredness in genetic counselling is mainly embedded in an ethos of non-directiveness, for which many reasons have been cited (e.g. Clarke 1997). Although non-directiveness remains the 'holy grail' of genetic counselling, debates continue about what exactly is meant by this term and its opposite. Kessler (1997, p.166) defines non-directiveness as 'procedures aimed at promoting the autonomy and self-directedness of the client'. Others (e.g. Fraser 1974; Sorenson 1993) characterize non-directiveness in terms of providing information and withholding advice; by extension, giving advice is equated with directiveness. Kessler (1997) considers coercion and persuasion, not advice-giving, as the core aspect of directiveness.

At another level, the ideal of non-directiveness as an attainable standard for genetic counselling practice also remains problematic. There is a recurrent call for a discontinuation of the 'pretense of neutrality' so counsellors acknowledge their moral responsibility as mediators of knowledge and facilitators of client decision-making (Stone and Miles 1999). Christopher (1996) argues that any counselling is inevitably underpinned by the professionals' 'moral visions'. A rigidly non-directive stance is said to run the risk of being perceived by vulnerable clients as a lack of responsiveness and of empathy, thus paradoxically posing a threat to client autonomy and resulting in the patient feeling a sense of being abandoned (Bosk 1992). Among others, Clarke (1991) rightly asks: 'is non-directiveness possible in genetic counselling?' With regard to prenatal screening and diagnosis, he claims that the social and psychological consequences of counselling make is impossible for clinical geneticists to adopt a non-directive stance. For instance, prenatal diagnosis consultations are bound to favour options of tests and termination. Moreover, the structure of the client counsellor encounter, especially involving various members of the family, does not facilitate a non-directive approach. As Clarke (1997, p.185) argues, 'giving priority to non-directiveness, in the negative sense of not influencing our clients, would then run counter to respect for informed decision-making'. 'Appropriate directiveness' – or what Wolff and Jung (1995) see as the use of an experiential approach that acknowledges counselling as a process of influence in the Rogerian sense – is a more realistic expectation.

A further level concerns the evidence from empirically grounded studies about directive/non-directive counselling practice. Survey-style studies such as Bartels et al. (1997) report the existence of a diverse range of attitudes among genetic professionals regarding directiveness and non-directiveness. In a communication-based study, Michie et al. (1997) emphasize that non-directiveness is often defined by what is *not* done rather than by what is done. Using ratings from consultation transcripts, they compared them with counsellor-reported and counselee-reported directiveness. Rated directiveness was defined as advice, expressed views about, or selective reinforcement of counsellees' behaviour, thought or emotions. Such unitary categorization of directiveness is problematic as it assumes a one-to-one form-function relationship in language use. The complex relationship between direct/indirect speech and its directive/non-directive force is relevant here (Benkendorf et al. 2001). Moreover, following Silverman (1997), it is difficult to demarcate, at the interactional level, what constitutes an advice-giving sequence and what might be denoted as information-as-advice. This raises the issue of separating facts and values with regard to language use. Information cannot be seen as value-neutral, so its situational introduction and framing by the counsellor influences the client's decision-making process and compromises the client's autonomy in the broader social context (Rentmeester 2001).

Client-centredness is problematic in the context of genetic counselling because it can be difficult to determine who the client is. Clienthood remains a dispersed notion as decisions about testing and decisions about disclosure of one's genetic status are fraught with psychological, social and moral dilemmas. Those who argue in favour of a client-centred genetic counselling agenda draw particular attention to the primacy of psychosocial dimensions of counselling (Kessler 1997; Weil 2000, 2003). However, socio-moral issues bordering on self–other relations are hard to exclude in a given counselling activity (Sarangi *et al.* in press).

Self–other relations take a particular mutation in genetic counselling because of the familial basis of genetic conditions, with different possible configurations as far as an individual's genetic status is concerned. A diagnosis of 'affected', 'at-risk' or 'carrier' status can have implications for offspring, siblings and even parents in terms of their genetic inheritance. Thus, the carrier status, which will not result in illness of self, demands the other-orientation *par excellence.*

The characterization of genetic counselling above – which requires professionals to be client-centred as well as non-directive, and clients also to be other-oriented – points to inevitable tensions. It highlights how the ideologies of client-centredness, non-directiveness and other-orientation are manifest ecologically and discoursally at the level of situated counselling practice. Are the embedded values that make up this constellation compatible? Parsons' (1952) characterization of professional rationality in terms of 'functional specificity' and 'affective neutrality' presents us with a paradox: while 'functional specificity' underscores client-orientedness of a profession, 'affective neutrality' potentially signifies a profession's distanced, non-directive mode of operation, almost bordering on indifference towards the client. It raises the question: can professional neutrality and client-centredness be reconciled with professional authority and client autonomy in situated professional–client encounters? The notion of professional neutrality may be ideologically invested with regard to the provider–client relationship. In reality, the greater the shift towards client-centredness, the more likely it is that professional neutrality is compromised. This may be particularly so when patients exercise their rights and autonomy, foregrounding preferred expectations that may not align with professional or institutional agendas.

It is relevant to revisit the observation made by Shlien and Zimring (1966) in the context of psychotherapy research and practice in the 1960s:

[T]he shift from *non-directive* to *client-centred*...is not incidental revision of nomenclature. It signifies the clarification of a perspective... In the second decade of development, it became increasingly clear that *non-directive* is a negative term, a protest contra to *directive*, and misleading in that it merely suggests the absence of direction... In this shift the image of the therapist changes from that of the mirror-like, passively non-influencing listener to that of the sensitive, actively understanding human respondent. What is relevant to research is the way in which this shift in terminology is related to changing assumptions about the therapist's *activity*, with corresponding changes in research interests. When the therapist was viewed as essentially neutral, passive, self-effacing, all therapists would be assumed to be equal, i.e., homogeneous by virtue of their inactivity. When the therapist image changes, the research and theory tend to focus somewhat upon him, though still largely on the client. (p.426; emphasis in original)

It is noteworthy that professional and scholarly debates about paradigms such as client-centredness and non-directiveness tend to focus on what the therapist/counsellor should embody in practice. What is particularly salient in the above quotation is how a shift from non-directiveness to client-centredness amounts to tolerance of variability in counselling/ therapy practice as a means of staying within 'the client's complex, shifting, and internal frame of reference', thus moving away from an 'objective' biomedical model of intervention.

THE SELF–OTHER DYNAMICS: A THEORETICAL PERSPECTIVE

Central to both non-directiveness and client-centredness is the concept of self–other relationship. In theoretical terms I draw on Mead's characterization of self–other dynamics and suggest a three-part taxonomy, i.e. 'self-vs.-other', 'self-as-other' and 'self-and-other' (Sarangi 2007), in order to examine how counsellors and clients integrate (or not) co-present and absent family members into decisions about testing and decisions about disclosure of test results.

It is commonplace to juxtapose self and other in a self-vs.-other relation as is the case in the characterization of the 'cultural other', reflected in the us-vs.-them ideology. A point of departure would be a conceptualization of the self in terms of the other that stresses the relational orientation. For Mead (1967), as for Merleau-Ponty (1968), 'self' is a socially situated reflexive process, which is made possible through the perception of alterity. According to Mead (1967):

> It is by means of reflexiveness – the turning-back of the experience of the individual upon himself – that the whole social process is thus brought into the experience of the individuals involved in it. (p.134)

Mead's argument is based on a complex characterization of the 'I–me' distinction. The 'me' is the objectification of 'I', i.e. the 'I' is the active agent while the 'me' is the retrospective experience. The I–me relation thus indexes a dialogic notion of the self. The 'I' conceives itself as another would conceive it by 'taking the attitude of the other'. The 'me' symbolically represents the point of view of the community as a whole.

The 'I–me' dynamics can be extended to the counselling setting. The decisions a client makes may come across as I-actions, without much reflection on 'me' as 'others would see it', from another perspective. The counsellor's/therapist's role then becomes one of filling this gap, in encouraging reflection, both retrospectively and prospectively – almost like holding the mirror as the carer does to the child, to borrow and extend the metaphor from Merleau-Ponty (1968). In a sense, such an approach fuses intra- and inter-subjectivity, and aligns with the Buberian (1958) perspective on 'I' as relational in his 'I–Thou' relationship. The 'self-as-other' position is distinguishable from that of 'self-vs.-other'.

In Mead, the anticipatory responses are about 'the generalized other', rather than specific others. In the genetic counselling setting, both the generalized and the specific 'others' are at play as the 'common good' and individual family members become invoked. The specific 'other' can be extended to include third parties such as partners and other family members in the sense of 'self-and-other'.

In what follows, using the method of discourse analysis,[1] I explore the self–other dynamics in genetic counselling by paying particular

---

1   I adopt a broad notion of discourse analysis, centred around the multi-functional, context-specific nature of language use both in written texts and in spoken interaction. If we view discourse as both activity and account, then a central tenet of discourse analysis is the categorization of actions, intentions, characters, events, etc. in terms of linguistic, interactional (e.g. turn-taking) and rhetorical features (see Roberts and Sarangi 2005; Sarangi in press).

attention to the above-mentioned tensions between non-directiveness and client-centredness. The genetic counselling protocol in the UK encourages family members to attend clinic sessions and participate in the decision-making process. When family members are present, they need to be interactionally integrated into the decision-making process. When family members are not co-present in the clinic session, the counsellor routinely introduces the 'family-as-other' perspective. I will analyse two contrasting conditions[2] – breast cancer (BC) and Huntington's Disease (HD) – in two contrasting genetic counselling settings, one where the partner is absent (BC), and the other where the client's partner is present (HD).

THE ABSENT OTHER: THE CASE OF BREAST CANCER

The following case is taken from a breast cancer clinic, where the client (AF) attends the clinic on her own. It therefore becomes crucial for the genetic counsellor (G4) to find out about her partner's perspective and to do so via AF's reported accounts. G4 has previously asked the client (AF) what kinds of issues she is aware of in relation to testing and AF has mentioned her concern about the possibility of her children carrying the gene, with the implicit suggestion that she is undergoing testing for her children's sake – a very common reason shared by many clients. AF is also concerned about her own individual wellbeing.

Data example 1a[3]

01. G4 right (2.0).hh right well so so from <u>your</u> point of view the having presymptomatic testing is going to affect you personally (.) surgically

02. AF y-yes (.) if it turns out *(like that)*

03. G4 and also (.) um (.) implications for your children

04. AF *yeah* (.) I mean I thought I'd wait to discuss that (.) you know when (.) when I have the result

05. G4 yeah (.) er and I think that's sensible and that's the approach that we often take with other people and again it doesn't have to be because some people with younger children will have discussed it already

---

2   These conditions are contrastive in terms of availability/non-availability of therapeutic intervention. While breast cancer allows the possibility of intervention in the form of mastectomy, there is no cure/intervention for Huntington's Disease.

3   See Appendix 1 at the end of this chapter for transcription conventions, which have been simplified for the purposes of this book.

First, G4 summarises the client's reasons for testing and then introduces the perspective of the familial other by mentioning 'implications for your children'. AF justifies her future other-orientation in relation to disclosure of test results, while keeping her current decision to test as self-oriented. Another dimension of otherness is manifest, in turn 05, when G4 positively evaluates AF's position ('that's sensible') by underscoring the shared counselling protocol involving other people in similar situations, including 'some people with younger children...' Although at the surface-level, this strategy may appear to be client-centred and non-directive, the endorsement of what other people do (not) do at strategic interactional moments can direct counsellees towards a course of action preferred by the counsellor (Pilnick 2002). Whether this is persuasive coercion, or simply information that can exert some influence on clients' subsequent course of action, remains debatable.

Discussion about testing protocol routinely includes attention to consequences of testing, including the possibility of being confronted with unfavourable test results. In the next extract, we notice the self-and-other aspects being elaborated further, as AF is urged to think about future consequences following a hypothetical positive test result.

Data example 1b

01. G4 = how you would feel (.) if you'd been tested and had a positive gene result (.) you had faced with surgery (.) and you then had surgery (.) you know these are the series of events and (.) is it that you would prefer to live with (.) the possibility of (.) being fifty percent risk (.) and continue having surgery oh sorry continue thinking about testing yourself (.) or even the surgery (and) just thinking about fifty percent risk or (.) do you definitely want to know (1.0) with all the potential (.) impact of that (.) and especially having two children (.) how does it make you feel (.) as a mother (.) potentially having passed on (.) um the genetic alteration to to one of them [(.)] um (.) and these are all =

02. AF [mm]

03. G4 = sorts of personal issues and different people handle them completely differently and I can't (.) I can't predict how you will respond it's only you know how you will think about them but I can raise those issues that you really ought to think about (.) you ought to sit down (.) if it's easier talk about it with somebody else or write it down (.) but some but but they need to be (.) tackled before (^^^) or thought about

---

04. AF (2.0) *I (hav^^^^about)
05. G4 yep (1.0) I mean are there any issues that you'd want to (talk about ^^)
06. AF er I (.) presume I could have reconstruction of the breast surgery
07. N3 mm
08. G4 yes
09. N3 u-g- (.) and certainly if that was (.) um an avenue you wanted to pursue then (.) you know we have very close links with Breast Care

In turn 01, G4 first takes into account AF's individual concerns before orienting her to think of her 'other' role as a mother. The consequences of genetic testing for the family are foregrounded, thus positioning G4 in a potentially influential role. AF needs to take time to discuss and reflect on possible implications of her actions. In turn 03, G4 makes a concession by suggesting that 'different people handle issues completely differently'. This is a way of emphasizing client autonomy, i.e. AF can choose her own course of action. Note, however, the language of directness ('ought to') with regard to undertaking reflective thinking, as it urges the client to engage in a dialogue with an 'other'. Unlike the invoking of 'what others do' in the extract in Data example 1a (whereby modelling one's action along others is emphasized), here 'what others do' is mentioned to underline context-sensitive differences leading to different action pathways, which amounts to G4 being both client-centred and non-directive. In turn 05, AF is invited to approach the issue of testing from all angles. AF, however, is inclined to adopt an interventionist stance centred around herself if tested positive – 'I could have reconstruction of the breast surgery' (turn 06). This self-orientation is met with a reluctant approval from G4 and N3, marked first with minimal responses, and then followed by an offer of supportive referral to Breast Care, which underscores client-centredness.

In the next extract, towards the end of the session, G4 directly elicits the perspective of AF's partner (MP).

Data example 1c
10. G4 I'm fairly certain I dealt with all of the main (.) issues (3.0) I mean I guess the (.) some of the things I I m-sort of touched upon it (.) erm (.) I-in mentioning that we would prefer ((MP)) to be here as well but I guess the o-the other issues to be thinking about from your point of view are (.) I m-how much have you discussed it (1.0) with him (1.0)
11. AF um? (0.5) I've told him what I'm going to do ((slight laugh))

12. G4 yep
13. N3 is he supportive?
14. AF I think so (.) [yeah]
15. G4 [[yep
16. N3 [[mm
17. G4 so the (.) sort of (.) other questions I would (.) throw back at you are (.) um hopefully that's not being too (mean to put) are (.) are one how do you think (.) he feel <u>he</u> would approach you if you were found to carry the (^^^) alteration (.) and two if you did carry it how do you think he would feel in relation to you having (^^^^^) mastectomies as a course >>I mean that's<<
18. AF I think he'd think it was a sensible thing to do in the [circumstances]
19. G4 [yep] (1.0) and the (.) potential impact of it on your (.) relationship (0.5) together and obviously in that context (.) not beating about the bush I mean there are potential impacts um sexually as [well] (.) um (.) I'm not saying =
20. AF [*mm*]
21. G4 = that because I want to (^^^) all issues but I mean I'm just not wanting to ignore it as a potential um [(fact)]
22. AF [um] well <u>IF</u> I test positive that is something we'll have to [discuss]
23. G4 [yeah]
24. AF (^^^^^^^) till I've had the result of the test done I wouldn't (1.0) I don't feel the need to discuss it till I've had the result
25. G4 no yep which I think is (^^^^^^^^^)

In turn 01, G4 signals the preference for MP to be co-present as that would ensure the voicing of the other perspective. As the second best option, G4 then directly elicits MP's viewpoint. AF gives a minimalist, matter-of-fact response: 'I've told him what I'm going to do' (turn 02). This response fails to display MP's perspective, except that he has been informed of AF's actions, which leads to N3's direct question – 'is he supportive?' (turn 04). Here other-orientation takes the upper hand to ascertain whether the decision to test and the consequent therapeutic options following the test results is shared.

AF's response to N3's direct question – 'I think so' (05) – is a tentative one, framed in hypothetical thought format rather than the actual reporting of MP's stance. G4 then goes on to elaborate by breaking down the issues in hand into two parts (turn 08), requiring specific responses. In turn 10, we have evidence of 'appropriate directiveness' on G4's part to raise issues that may not have been taken into consideration by AF, and this could potentially influence both the decision to test and the surgical action following a positive test result. Following Shiloh (1996), we can interpret this as an instance of helping clients to make a decision wisely rather than making a (particular) 'wise' decision. Once again, MP's stance is presented in hypothetical language, which suggests that AF has not yet sought MP's reactions to her chosen course of action and that only a positive test result will necessitate the other-oriented dialogue.

THE CO-PRESENT OTHER: THE CASE OF HUNTINGTON'S DISEASE

Decision about testing can be motivated by a number of factors, ranging from future reproductive options to protect children and grandchildren from inheriting the genetic condition to knowing one's genetic status *per se*. Knowing for the sake of others is perhaps most pronounced in the case of predictive testing for Huntington's Disease (HD).[4] My next case concerns a client (AF) who is at risk of HD. AF is in her mid-60s at the time of recording the sessions. Although her mother, now deceased, was diagnosed with HD some 30 years ago, AF had not tested herself then because of the lack of availability of genetic testing. Only recently AF began to consider the option of testing in light of her maternal aunt being diagnosed with HD, and her own grandchildren coming of age. AF's own children are very much against her having the test as they are worried that a positive test result, which is likely, could be very distressing for AF. By contrast, AF anticipates a negative test result on which to anchor her other-orientation: 'the best thing I could ever give them [grandchildren] is to send them a bouquet and say everything is fine (.) that it no longer has to be told to any of the younger grandchildren'. Her responsibility to terminate the uncertainty about the genetic transmission down the family line is the key motivating factor for AF's decision to undergo testing. AF is accompanied on each of her clinic visits by her partner (MP), whose perspective is directly elicited by the genetic counsellor (G5) in the extract below.

---

4   Huntington's Disease is a late-onset, degenerative neuropsychiatric disorder, with no effective treatment. Predictive tests are, however, available, which can attest that there is a 50% chance that the child of an affected parent will have inherited the disease-associated mutation.

Data example 2a

01. G5: so mister ((MP)) I mean how do you feel about the issue of testing particularly when things [(^^^)]

02. MP: [I] am fully with ((AF)) if she wants to do it (1.5) so be it (.) we'll accept that but (1.0) I don't want the family wants her to do it (.) and we we would like your advice if that's possible (1.0)

03. G5: mm

04. MP: either to or not

05. AF: I think one thing for certain is that when ((N2)) told us that the blood could be [...]

In response to G5's direct question, MP displays his other-orientation by stressing that he is happy to accept AF's decision as long as it is done for her own sake rather than for the family's sake, thus indexing a self-vs.-other stance. The family-other is kept at a distance so as not to compromise client autonomy. Strategically, MP turns this opportunity to an advice-seeking one, but G5 is not forthcoming with any direct advice (see G5's minimal response 'mm' in turn 03, and no response immediately following turn 04).

In the next extract, AF continues with her account of not letting her children know about the testing process and wonders if she is doing the right thing, thus seeking direct advice from G5.

Data example 2b

01. AF: yes I think er (.) it it's just something that's (.) I I haven't even mentioned this to ((MP)) it's just something that run through my mind and I thought well (.) I might just as well ask now because (.) we've never kept secrets in the family (.) and it's something that doesn't come easy (.) to me to do (1.0) hhh (.) I'm trying to shield my children in [one] way

02. G5: [mm]

03. AF: and would I be doing the right thing (1.0) I don't know (1.0) 'cause they are most certainly dead against me having the test done (1.5) they both are (1.5) and my son is most (.) certainly

04. G5: *mm* (1.0)

05. AF: isn't he? ((to MP))
    ((MP nods))

06. AF: he just says we're opening a can or worms (1.0) by doing it

07. G5: because it's the possibility=

08. AF: =of it being positive (.) yes

09. G5: (^^^^^^^)

---

10. AF: mm
    (1.0)
11. MP: so you can appreciate the dilemma [that we are in] although
    ((AF's)) it's =
12. G5: [it is it is a true dilemma]
13. MP: = (.) a at the end of the day it's ((AF's)) decision
14. G5: mhm
15. MP: and I fall in (with that) (1.0) but we would like your advice
16. G5: in terms of (attending for) the process (..) it's not unusual for
    people to do that without particularly telling very many people that
    they're going through it
17. AF: mm
18. G5: people actually will go through the process without informing
    close relatives because of all the anxiety that's around (.) it's difficult
    (.) knowing that everybody else knows when you're coming for your
    interviews
19. AF: yes
20. G5: it's difficult knowing that everybody else knows when you're
    coming for the test [and] when the result's due so it's not unusual (.)
    for people to sort of =
21. AF: [yes]
22. G5: = (.) hide that process (1.0) I think that's a different issue from
    hiding the result

AF advances the other-oriented 'shielding the children' as the main reason behind her decision to keep the test-process a family secret. She formulates it as a moral dilemma – 'would I be doing the right thing' – and further heightens it through the reported speech of her son – 'we are opening a can of worms' (turn 06). MP once again remains other-oriented with regard to AF's decision-making, while seeking direct advice from G5. As before, G5 does not offer any direct advice, but draws on his/ her clinical experience of what other people do in these circumstances, thereby implying his/her preference about the decision itself (turn 16). This choice to introduce information about what others do therefore cannot be seen as value-neutral. The client-centred orientation, however, is evident as both AF and MP want to be assured that what they are doing to manage the testing process is 'not unusual'. In turns 18–20, G5 alludes to the possibility of keeping the testing process a guarded secret. Again, based on clinical experience of other cases, G5 indicates that the timing of disclosure is often problematic, which may lead to hiding the testing process, unlike the test result itself (turn 22). By incorporating what is usual, i.e. what other people do, G5 strategically balances his client-centredness with a rather dubious non-directive stance.

As part of the HD protocol, and prior to proceeding with the testing procedure, it is routine practice for counsellors to initiate a discussion about the significance of test results for self and for others. Our final example is illustrative.

Data example 2c

01. G5: and I think (.) the discussion (has to be over) (.) if we go ahead with the test (.) what are we going to do (.) (when we have the results) (.) WHICH IS something that we're happy to talk through with you as part of the process (1.0) *(^^^^^^)* (.) as a couple

02. AF: how would you feel about it if I had it done that way ((to MP))

03. MP: ((slight laugh)) you can't put the onus [on me ((AF))]

04. AF: [NO no] BUT how how would you

05. MP: SOMETHING THAT I I wouldn't er=

06. AF: =HOW would you feel about it if it was done [that way]

07. MP: [I would] I would follow you w-whichever way you wanted it (2.0) y-you know my feelings [we've spoken] about this [time and time] and =

08. AF: [it's just this]

09. MP: = time (again)

10. AF: [it's just for p-] it's just for protection for my children that's (.) that's the only way that I'm lo-that's the only way that I can even (.) have this idea of (.) of keeping it secret
    (2.0)

11. G5: *mm*

12. AF: I mean if it came back and it was er everything was clear and positive well I mean we could shout it from the hill tops couldn't we to them ((laughing)) you know (.) but what if it's the other way (1.0) which I'm well aware of (1.0) quite well aware of that the that there is a possibility (1.0) because I'm fine I'm I'm not that (.) sure of myself that I can go into it and think it's going to come out that way (..) 'cause I'm not (2.0) I'm not (3.0) but I'm hh (.) I myself want to know and I'm trying to get around it (1.0)

13. G5: so whenever you think about it (.) whenever you go through all (..) the dilemmas involved in (what) you come back to (.) *is that you want to know*

14. AF: I would like to know (.) personally (.) I really would like to know

15. G5: *mm*

16. AF: myself (..) and I would (2.0) I felt this way when I was told and had time to calm down from it all (1.0) many times I kept saying to them I

---

wish there was a test I could have done (.) now (.) and that was after
the initial shock that wasn't just (.) being in shock and speaking about
it (.) and I would have gone there and then and had it done (2.0) I
know I went through a period of telling them no I didn't want to
know (.) which you do (.) as if but at this time now yes I would (0.3) I
would like to know

17. G5: *mm* (1.0) so in a sense the issue is what what do you do with
the result really

18. AF: yes (1.0) yes (1.0) that would be the issue (0.2) not the fact of
having it (.) having the test (..)

19. G5: and that in a sense does come down to the two possibilities
which is that you tell them (.) *or you (.) you hold it back and keep it
a secret*

20. AF: mhm
(1.0)

21. G5: *(^^^) (.) 'cause you've met the whole family ((N2)) haven't you*
(1.0)

22. N2: *yeah.* (.) I guess the trouble with it's back to the trouble with
secrets is someone always finds out and then you have to deal with
the

23. AF: *mm*

24. N2: the backlash

25. AF: mm

26. N2: (and that) (..) um (0.2) you have to deal with the backlash of
perhaps going through it all without anyone knowing as well (..) I
guess 'cause the (..)

27. AF: yeah

28. N2: I would imagine they would be upset with the thought that you
having done it and nobody knew

Following G4's framing of the post-test scenario for reflection, in a
rather unusual fashion, AF attempts to bring MP into the discussion
directly ('how would you feel about it if I had it done that way', turn
02). MP is taken by surprise with the spotlight directed at him and
his opinion, as can be seen from his embarrassed laughter. But what
follows is a directive line of questioning on AF's part, which coerces MP
to declare his unfailing support for AF's decision – an endorsement of
testing for AF's own sake and of keeping the testing procedure a family
secret. It is noteworthy that G5 facilitates the ongoing self-and-other
discussion between AF and MP by maintaining an interactional silence
in a non-directive fashion. In turn 10, once again AF orients herself to
the family-others ('it's just for protection of my children') as a way of

justifying her decision to keep the testing procedure a secret. AF then spells out her future response to the test results being, hypothetically, positive or negative (turn 12). In the event of a negative test result, the good news would be shared with the family loudly and publicly ('we could shout it from the hill tops'). If, however, it turned out to be a positive test result, it would call for quiet self-reflections. AF nonetheless considers a positive test result as an unlikely outcome as she says 'I'm not that (.) sure of myself that I can go into it and think it's going to come out that way', which aligns with her family-as-other orientation in her desire to free the grandchildren of any future anxiety. In turn 13, G5 returns to the core aspect of the decision for testing, i.e. the desire to know for oneself, which leads AF to admit that the decision process has been a long-winded one. The formulation 'I would have gone there and then' (turn 16) takes us back to the position AF occupied in the past ('I went through a period of telling them no I don't want to know') which is contrasted with her position in the present ('but at this time now yes I would like to know').

In turns 17 and 19, G5 shifts the topic to dissemination of test results and goes on to offer various available options in the spirit of non-directiveness, including the possibility of keeping secrets within the family. At this point G5 directly invites N2 to voice an opinion, given that the latter was involved in the home visit (turn 21). Having met the whole family, N2 seems to be in a position to bring in their perspectives to potentially influence the decision-making process. As we can see, N2 warns against family secrets in a matter-of-fact way by appealing to realistic consequences that can follow a leakage, which cannot be ruled out. She also draws attention to further consequences of such leakage – the backlash that might force the family to go through the testing procedure once again as if it had never happened before (data not shown), thus causing unnecessary upset. This prospective scenario-building endorses, in a directive manner, the disfavoured option of keeping secrets from family members.

CONCLUSIONS

In this chapter my main concern has been to illustrate the ways in which competing professional values are manifest at a micro-level in professional–client encounters, as well the extent to which they impact upon clients. As far as clients are concerned, there are many competing tensions in genetic counselling – decision about genetic testing for one's own sake *vis-à-vis* children's and/or grandchildren's sake; going through the testing process by entertaining a negative test result as the most likely outcome; the motivation for hiding the testing process from other family members in order to avoid unwarranted anxiety; the decision about when it would be right to disclose what to whom; assuming an 'as if normal' self to hide the counselling process, etc. The tensions can be linked to withholding the truth to 'shield' other family members, as we saw in the second case concerning Huntington's Disease. In both cases, the clients adopt the utilitarian perspective by foregrounding a commonsense approach while considering the weighting of consequences of disclosure in relation to a definitive time-frame.

The genetic professionals are, no doubt, caught in this web of clients' justifications and excuses (Scott and Lyman 1968) in the sense that evaluation of current and future states of affairs resulting from disclosure and non-disclosure is an integral part of their accounts/decisions. While the complexity of the concerns raised is easy to identify in the situated accounts, it is harder to establish any hierarchical relation between the competing modes of reasoning that drive the individual actions/decisions in specific instances. At a reflective level, genetic counsellors routinely introduce their impressions about other people's experience as a way of providing a basis for enabling the 'I–me' dialogue (Buber 1958), i.e. to encourage clients to take the other perspectives into account. This often leads to a directive stance with regard to a procedure of reflection rather than a proposal for a particular course of action (Shiloh 1996). However, incorporating into the talk what others do similarly or differently does underscore a value position.

In genetic counselling, both counsellors and clients have to be other-oriented by 'decentring the client' and a balance between 'self' and 'other' somehow needs to be struck. The counsellor – by seeking the family-as-other perspectives, and by incorporating what people-as-other 'normally' do – becomes other-oriented in a directive sense. This stance on the part of the counsellor ultimately makes the client other-oriented. Such a stance conflates the 'self-vs.-other', 'self-as-other' and 'self-and-other' positions. It also draws our attention to the existence of many different 'others' whose perspectives must count in the decision-making process.

Against this backdrop, the dynamic relationship between directiveness, non-directiveness and client-centredness needs revisiting, with further systematic analysis of the 'black box' of genetic counselling discourse by paying particular attention to the context-specificity of various genetic conditions. When therapeutic intervention is feasible, as in the case of breast cancer, the counsellor adopting a directive stance may be appropriate. Also, when it is a matter of involving other family members in the decision-making process where no therapeutic intervention is available, as in HD, it may be desirable for counsellors to ask clients directly about who is included in and/or excluded from such decision-making without necessarily passing evaluation about what is right or wrong in a given family sphere.

APPENDIX 1: TRANSCRIPTION CONVENTIONS

(.) (..): micropause up to one second
(1.0, 2.0): pause timed in seconds
CAPITAL LETTERS: increased volume
word: decreased volume
underlining: increased emphasis as in stress
question mark [?]: rising intonation
-: cut-off of prior word or sound
[text in square brackets]: overlapping speech
((text in double round brackets)): description or anonymized information
(text in round brackets): transcriber's guess
(^^^^^^): untranscribable
=: a continuous utterance

RESPONSE
Heather Skirton

Srikant Sarangi has skilfully highlighted some of the conflicting pressures inherent in the practice of genetic counselling, showing how the subtle turns in discourse can exert influences on both the client and the counsellor. The major issue from my perspective is the potential conflict between maintaining professional distance and promoting client-centredness.

One of the original core values of genetic counselling was non-directiveness. It may be that embedding the principle of non-directiveness into genetic counselling was a response to the eugenic practices in a number of countries that ranged along a spectrum from 'positive eugenics' that included encouraging those of 'good stock' to reproduce (supported by the Eugenics Society in England in the first part of the twentieth century), to negative eugenics, the elimination of those not considered worthy of life in our society as practised under the Nazi regime in Germany. However, the establishment of specialist genetic services also coincided with the rise of modernism, a concept embodying the right to self-determination and autonomy and it is likely that this also had an impact.

Whatever its origins, non-directiveness became the mantra of genetic counsellors, first in the US and then in Europe, so that in the 1990s genetic counsellors were committed to a style of consultation in which they declined to offer guidance. Indeed, to advise clients on a course of action was deemed incompetent. Although originally a proponent of non-directiveness (Kessler 1979), Seymour Kessler was forced to challenge the interpretation of the term by genetic counsellors, stating that it should mean freedom from coercion rather than a communicative vacuum (Kessler 1997).

Carl Rogers, the founder of person-centred counselling espoused the view that everyone is capable of deciding the route that is best for themselves (Rogers 1961). In the case of genetic counselling, then, clients are capable of making the best possible decisions for their own lives. However, they may lack the confidence to do this, especially if attuned to a paternalistic health care system. The skill of the counsellor lies in facilitating the clients in making their own decisions by reinforcing self-belief. In terms of the discourse of a genetic counselling consultation, it appears to me that Sarangi has not mentioned a factor that could have a significant impact in this regard. As there are some situations in which clients can only be involved in shared decision-making with the appropriate input of the counsellor, on whom they rely to provide the necessary expertise (Emery 2001; van Zwieten *et al.* 2006), a non-directive approach by the counsellor could result in a frustrating dialogue for both parties. While counsellors may see their role as one that enhances client autonomy, clients may not necessarily differentiate between a 'usual' medical encounter (in which advice and guidance are freely offered) and the genetic consultation. The dichotomous nature of expectations could lead to disruption to the verbal discourse before it begins. In my clinical experience, the philosophical basis to the genetic counselling encounter is not explicitly discussed with clients, except in those situations where the client directly asks for advice. Only then are they told that the counsellor is not prepared to give advice. In some circumstances the counsellor may decline to comment further; however, a skilled counsellor will go on to support the client in exploring the best route for themselves.

While information is not value-neutral, clients are often in unknown territory (Skirton 2001) and may seek assurance that what they are considering is not unusual. There is an additional conflict that arises in practice with respect to professional neutrality. If the client expresses a value or belief that clearly demonstrates they do not consider a course of action acceptable, should the counsellor provide further information (for example, on the option of termination of pregnancy) on the grounds that they are compromising their professional neutrality by not doing so? I would argue that client-centredness is infinitely more facilitative than professional neutrality, even if that exists.

Of course, human beings bring their own beliefs and attitudes into every encounter. In a genetic counselling consultation, the counsellor, as well as the client, will bring their core values. This is not wrong, but in order to work effectively in the helping professions, it is essential to be non-judgemental. The majority of those working in genetics do not have a strong basic training in counselling skills, and I would argue that one of the main purposes of such training is to enable the practitioner to hold the client in high regard, to have belief in the client's ability to decide for themselves and to make the counsellor aware of his or her own issues and how they intrude into the consultation. Sarangi's chapter illuminates the ways in which even supposedly subtle exchanges can convey the counsellor's, as well as the client's, underlying beliefs. Clarke (1997) suggests that adopting a non-directive stance helps the counsellor to establish an appropriate emotional distance from the client, but this also has the impact of reducing the empathic relationship between the parties and it would be preferable if counsellors were enabled to maintain psychological boundaries in the context of an empathic relationship, through training and supervision.

In the examples Sarangi used, the counsellors' own issues persisted in being heard, despite attempts at non-directiveness. This creates dissonance in the counsellor that precludes genuine communication. In the first case the counsellor seemed worried about the client having a mastectomy, emphasizing the husband's role in the decision and potential 'sexual' difficulties. In the second, the wish of the client to keep her test secret was obviously uncomfortable for the counsellor. In these cases, perhaps the counsellor uses the 'what others do' device to present their own views in a more acceptable (to them) form. I suggest in both cases the client and counsellor may have left the encounter dissatisfied.

I find Sarangi's assertion that a counsellor will tend to see testing and termination as the preferable pathway for those seeking prenatal counselling interesting, as this implies that counsellors have an agenda connected with the use of technology to help couples to avoid the births of affected children. I am not convinced that counsellors really do have an agenda that promotes the use of testing: experienced practitioners will be aware that technology creates, as well as solves, human problems. I would also question whether it is more acceptable to be directive when an intervention is available that may prevent or ameliorate a problem. If autonomy is considered an important concept, the autonomous right to make a decision should not be dependent on the impact of the decision on the individual. Providing the person is appropriately informed of the implications, any decision should be acceptable, even if the counsellor believes it puts the client at greater risk of harm. For health professionals, however, an outcome that may result in diminished wellbeing for the client may be perceived as a failure – and an outcome that may expose the health professional to criticism or even litigation.

In the examples given, it appears that the counsellors tend further towards a client-centred approach than towards professional neutrality. Sarangi identifies the way in which the counsellor reflects the 'me' perspective, to bring the client's attention to the ways in which his or her actions might be seen from the viewpoint of the 'other'. However, there may also be situations where the client focuses so much on the 'other' that the counsellor is concerned that he or she has failed to acknowledge the impact on themselves. In this case, the counsellor may feel obliged to advocate for the client's 'self'.

In conclusion, I agree that non-directiveness in the context of genetic counselling is a value that is past its 'use by date'. Valuable communication is based on the genuineness of both parties and a non-judgemental approach – characteristics of the interaction that may enhance the client's ability to make a decision wisely (Shiloh 1996). While many new questions are raised by the application of discourse analysis to the genetic counselling encounter, we have yet to find many of the answers.

REFERENCES

Bartels, D.M., LeRoy, B.S., McCarthy, P. and Caplan, A.L. (1997) 'Non-directiveness in genetic counseling: a survey of practitioners.' *American Journal of Medical Genetics 72*, 2, 172–179.

Benkdenorf, J.L., Prince, M.B., Rose, M.A., De Fina, A. and Hamilton, H.E. (2001) 'Does indirect speech promote non-directive genetic counselling? Results of a sociolinguistic investigation.' *American Journal of Medical Genetics 106*, 3, 199–207.

Bosk, C. (1992) *All God's Mistakes: Genetic Counseling in a Paediatric Clinic.* Chicago: The University of Chicago Press.

Buber, M. (1958) *I and Thou.* Edinburgh: T. and T. Clark.

Christopher, J.C. (1996) 'Counselling's inescapable moral visions.' *Journal of Counselling and Development 75* (Sept/Oct), 17–25.

Clarke, A. (1991) 'Is non-directive genetic counselling possible?' *Lancet 338*, 8773, 998–1001.

Clarke, A. (1997) 'The Process of Genetic Counselling: Beyond Non-directiveness.' In P.S. Harper and A.J. Clarke (eds) *Genetics, Society and Clinical Practice.* Oxford: Bios Scientific Publishers.

Emery, J. (2001) 'Is informed choice in genetic testing a different breed of informed decision-making? A discussion paper.' *Health Expectations 4*, 2, 81–86.

Fraser, F.C. (1974) 'Genetic counselling.' *American Journal of Human Genetics 26*, 5, 636–659.

Illich, I. (1977) 'Disabling Professions.' In I. Illich with I.K. Zola, J. McNight, J. Caplan and H. Shaiken (eds) *Disabling Professions.* London: Marion Boyars.

Kessler, S. (1979) 'The psychological foundations of genetic counselling.' In S. Kessler (ed.) *Genetic Counselling: Psychological Dimensions.* New York: Academic Press.

Kessler, S. (1997) 'Psychological aspects of genetic counselling. xi. Non-directiveness revisited.' *American Journal of Medical Genetics 72*, 2, 164–171.

Mead, G.H. (1967, first published 1934) *Mind, Self and Society.* Chicago, IL: University of Chicago Press.

Merleau-Ponty, M. (1968) *The Primacy of Perception and Other Essays.* Evanston, IL: Northwestern University Press.

Michie, S., Bron, F., Bobrow, M. and Marteau, T.M. (1997) 'Non-directiveness in genetic counseling: an empirical study.' *American Journal of Human Genetics 60*, 1, 40–47.

Parsons, T. (1952) *The Social System.* London: Tavistock.

Pilnick, A. (2002) 'What "most people" do: exploring the ethical implications of genetic counselling.' *New Genetics and Society 21*, 3, 339–350.

Rentmeester, C.A. (2001) 'Value neutrality in genetic counselling: an unattained ideal.' *Medicine, Health Care and Philosophy 4*, 1, 47–51.

Roberts, K. and Sarangi, S. (2005) 'Theme-oriented discourse analysis of medical encounters.' *Medical Education 39*, 632–640.

Rogers, C. (1951) *Client-Centred Therapy: Its Current Practice, Implications and Theory.* Boston, MA: Houghton Mifflin.

Rogers, C. (1961) *On Becoming a Person: A Therapist's View of Psychotherapy.* London: Constable.

Sarangi, S. (2000) 'Activity Types, Discourse Types and Interactional Hybridity: The Case of Genetic Counselling.' In S. Sarangi and M. Coulthard (eds) *Discourse and Social Life.* London: Pearson.

Sarangi, S. (2007) 'Other-orientation in Patient-centred Health Care Communication: Unveiled Ideology or Discoursal Ecology?' In G. Garzone and S. Sarangi (eds) *Discourse, Ideology and Ethics in Specialised Communication.* Berne: Peter Lang.

Sarangi, S. (in press) 'Practising Discourse Analysis in Healthcare Settings.' In I. Bourgeault, R. DeVries and R. Dingwall (eds) *Qualitative Methods in Health Research.* London: Sage.

Sarangi, S., Brookes-Howell, L., Bennert, K. and Clarke, A. (in press) 'Psychological and Sociomoral Frames in Genetic Counselling for Predictive Testing.' In C.N. Candlin and S. Sarangi (eds) *Communication in Professions and Organizations.* Berlin: Mouton de Gruyter.

Scott, M.B. and Lyman, S.M. (1968) 'Accounts.' *American Social Review 33*, 1, 46–62.

Shiloh, S. (1996) 'Decision-making in the Context of Genetic Risk.' In T. Marteau and M. Richards (eds) *The Troubled Helix: Social and Psychological Implications of the New Human Genetics.* Cambridge: Cambridge University Press.

Shlien, J.M. and Zimring, F.M. (1966) 'Research Directives and Methods in Client-centred Therapy.' In L.A. Gottschalk and A.H. Auerbach (eds) *Methods of Research in Psychotherapy.* New York: Appleton-Century-Crofts.

Silverman, D. (1997) *Discourses of Counselling: HIV Counselling as Social Interaction.* London: Sage.

Skirton, H. (2001) 'The client's perspective of genetic counseling – a grounded theory study.' *Journal of Genetic Counselling 10,* 4, 311–329.

Sorenson, J.R. (1993) 'Genetic Counselling: Values that Have Mattered.' In D. Bartels, B. LeRoy and A. Caplan (eds) *Prescribing Our Future: Ethical Challenges in Genetic Counselling.* New York: Aldine de Gruyter.

Stone, H.W. and Miles, R. (1999) 'Moral direction in genetic counselling: prenatal testing and Huntington's Disease.' *Families, Systems and Health 17,* 1, 75–87.

van Zwieten, M., Willems, D., Knegt, L. and Leschot, N. (2006) 'Communication with patients during the prenatal testing procedure: an explorative qualitative study.' *Patient Education and Counseling 63,* 1–2, 161–168.

Weil, J. (2000) *Psychosocial Genetic Counselling.* Oxford: Oxford University Press.

Weil, J. (2003) 'Psychosocial genetic counselling in the post-non-directive era: a point of view.' *Journal of Genetic Counselling 12,* 3, 199–211.

Wolff, G. and Jung, C. (1995) 'Non-directiveness and genetic counselling.' *Journal of Genetic Counselling 4,* 1, 3–25.

Chapter 9

The Chaplain's Dilemma

Paul Ballard

INTRODUCTION

One of the seeming paradoxes of the recent history of the National
Health Service (NHS) has been the growth in the number of chaplains
employed in the country's hospitals; 296 full time in 1990 increasing
to 354 in 1998 (Orchard 2000). Of course, the chaplains have a long
tradition behind them. At the same time, however, changes, both within
the health service and beyond, have brought increasing new threats and
pressures. Internally, the so-called 'modernization' of health provision
introduced major changes in the way the service is understood and
delivered, imposing financial constraints and, therefore, measured
targets and outcomes. Externally, there have been major social changes,
notably (in the context that we are currently discussing) the effects of
radical multi-culturalism and religious pluralism, together with a shift in
religious consciousness away from the traditional institutional forms to
a more diffuse yet widespread valuation of spirituality. Such movements
have inevitably affected hospital chaplaincies as they have had to find
creative ways of working in a large, publicly funded institution.

   This chapter attempts to look at some of the significant questions this
poses to health care chaplains. It will be done in two sections: a) the place
of the chaplaincy service within the NHS and its particular contribution
and the pressure to conform to the professional models found in health
care; b) the changes demanded by working in a multi-faith community
and the implications of the emergence of 'spiritual health' as part of the
healing process.

   It would be easy, because of their often marginalized position,
smallness of numbers and special concerns, to belittle the importance of

chaplains. However, what is happening to the chaplaincy service is not an isolated experience or peculiar to them. Their story very much represents what is happening at many key points within the NHS as a whole, not least in underlining some inherent contradictions in the strategic assumptions that lie behind current health care policies – placed as they are between the Scylla of cost-efficiency and technological advance and the Charybdis of the desire to offer holistic, personalized care.

CHAPLAINCY WITHIN THE NHS

It was always assumed, enshrined in the NHS at its foundation and recently reinforced by the Patients Charter in 1991 (McSherry 2006; Orchard 2001), that hospitals 'should give special attention to provide for the spiritual needs of both patients and staff' (un-attributed quote in Hospital Chaplain's Council 1978, p.6) This was primarily done by providing full- or part-time chaplains from the clergy of mainstream churches (the Church of England (C of E), the Catholic Church and the Free Churches) to be paid for from the health budget. Appointments were made by the area health authority in collaboration with the churches. Locally, there was to be a joint board for both the full-time and part-time posts, allocated according to a national formula relating to the numbers of those patients that claimed religious allegiance. Such appointments were to be made from clergy recognized by their denominations as suitable to provide this specialized ministry. Such clergy came under the aegis at national level, for the Anglicans and Free Churches, of the Joint Committee for Hospital Chaplaincies (serviced by the C of E) and, for the Catholics, the Bishops' Conference. There were similar arrangements for the Jewish community. In effect, therefore, clergy were seconded into the health service for a pastoral ministry that was regarded as a variant of the normal parish or congregational ministry. The NHS was 'buying in' a service and for many part-time and some full-time chaplains this literally meant that the churches were the financial beneficiary rather than the individual. For those clergy concerned their primary professional identity came from their ecclesiastical recognition. Only over time, did they begin to develop a sense of having a particular, 'sector' ministry and, therefore, to form their own 'guild'. A somewhat similar pattern can also be found with other health professionals, such as doctors, whose expertise was, to varying extents, bought in to the health service. This dual allegiance to one's professional body and to the NHS was for the chaplains, perhaps, more sharply drawn than for most since they were straddling two sets of institutional practice. Thus the health service was, in effect, an organizing structure that brought together the various professional groups as contributors to a common enterprise.

Recent developments

However, in recent years the 'managerial revolution' in the NHS has shifted the balance of authority away from the professions to the employing structures. Moreover, this has been moulded by models of management believed to be generic and therefore universally applicable, borrowed from commerce and industry. Stephen Pattison (1997) has described this as a move away from 'administration' to 'managerialism', which he describes as a mixture of 'neo-Taylorism' or 'neo-Drukerism' leavened with 'new wave' styles that use the language of 'motivation, flexibility, innovation, development, quality, getting close to the customer and so on' (p.22). But 'management by objectives' is predominantly about productivity, throughput and efficiency. The various elements that go to make up a complex institution are thus made subordinate to what is seen as its central mission: i.e. speedy, efficient and customer-led solutions to perceived health problems.

The immediate impact of this on the health care chaplains has been to bring them more firmly into the orbit of the health service and thus to accentuate their clerically professional distinctiveness:

> The Department of Health has only recently begun to 'own' its employment of chaplains through more active management. This represents a dramatic change in the formal conception of chaplaincy, with the chaplaincy 'departments' written about in the 1960s and 70s giving way to the 2003 guidance title of 'NHS Chaplaincy'. At a single stroke the health service demonstrates its intentions to house chaplains of all faiths within structures that claimed to make no doctrinal or theological judgement. (Swift 2004, p.5)

These guidelines appear to retain the traditional collaboration with the faith communities (now nationally represented by the Multi-faith Group for Health Care Chaplaincy), and even to enhance the position of chaplaincies in the NHS, but it does so by locking them into the new institutional management structures.

The recommended procedure is to identify a board-level director in a Trust to become an advocate for the chaplaincy-spiritual care team, who may or may not be a chaplain. That team is then expected to conform to the standard managerial practices as laid down for 'human resources' and 'lines of management/accountability' (Multi-faith Group for Health Care Chaplaincy 2003, p.8). This process of 'modernization' is further reinforced by the crucial report *Caring for the Spirit* (South Yorkshire Strategic Health Authority 2003), which seeks to map out a model that is customer-led and universally applicable regardless of faith and creed. It also advocates a much clearer professional career path within the chaplaincy service itself, thus reinforcing their position within the NHS. All this poses a real turning point in their identity – that is subject to considerable debate within both faith communities and chaplaincy organizations and which has not yet been resolved.

A further consequence of managerialism is the way in which it reinforces an already strongly present bias in the provision of health. Some time ago Bob Lambourne (1983) drew attention to the disproportionate weight given to the acute, high-tech end of health care, such as surgery, at the expense of the chronic, long-term, low-tech services such as geriatrics, mental health, preventative medicine or social welfare. The emphasis on productivity strengthens this. The chaplain is, however, among the second-class citizens at the Cinderella end of health care. Interestingly, this can lead chaplains to try to strengthen their position by working closely with the high-tech areas of medicine at the expense of care in long-stay units (Orchard 2000).

Implications for the chaplain's role

The trends described above raise a number of issues concerning, for example, the chaplain's position in the medical team. How far is or can the chaplain be drawn into the heart of the caring process? All too often it is a matter of waiting in the wings, to be called in on request, often to pick up the emotional pieces, or being regarded as an occasional visitor to the ward. This marginality is starkly underlined in the 2003 guidance, where it is stated that, because of the Data Protection Act, a patient's permission is specifically required before any medical information can be revealed to the chaplain rather than, as has been normal hitherto, the chaplain being included in the general agreement covering the medical team as a whole. Swift (2005) comments that the Patient Information Advisory Group do not perceive chaplains to be part of the care team to a degree that they can access information of a type available to other staff.

In part, among NHS managers anxiety may be about the range of people involved, i.e. full-time and part-time chaplains and lay volunteers, and their professional standing. But such restrictions can be disastrous to the way the chaplain works, confining him/her to those who specifically ask for their help and even blocking the possibility of general ward rounds unless invited by every patient there. It can also hamper pastoral relations if the chaplain does not have reasonable access to information. It is ironic that this concern has been raised in relation to a profession that has, in law, the right to client confidentiality.

There is another ambiguity that should be noted here. Hospital chaplains have always had a 'twin track' brief: to both patients and staff. The second task can primarily be understood as being available to support hard-pressed nurses, doctors and others, especially, perhaps, when they are facing acute moral dilemmas; but there is also a longstanding tradition that the chaplain is there for the wellbeing of the institution as such. This requires a certain level of independence and distance from the system while at the same time being embedded in it. A well-known analogy for this was Heije Faber's image of the clown as found in the mediaeval court (Faber 1971). The clown is present everywhere but belongs to nowhere. The clown is free to approve or disapprove without fear or favour, though he can be kicked or ignored. Indeed, evidence suggests that what is valued by the patients and staff is someone who is available on the edge of the system, with whom one can talk freely without any agenda or consequences (Ballard et al. 1999, 2000; Wilson 1971). Hospital chaplains, however, are at present being more and more firmly regarded as employees of the NHS rather than of the churches (similar to prison chaplains), with all that that means in terms of institutional loyalty.

This sense of being a stranger within the service, however, has allowed the chaplain to represent and articulate (by implication if not always aloud) such questions as: 'What is a hospital for?'; 'What makes for good health?'; 'How best do we value the human being?' Any institution, especially one so close to basic human needs, will inevitably embody certain assumptions, values and understandings of what it means to be human and the good of society, many of which will reflect those of the wider community. Perhaps it is the chaplain's special task to be, in this sense, what every institution needs: a devil's advocate or the grit in the oyster.

This can be illustrated by reference to Michael Wilson's (1971) typology. He suggests there are four aspects of a hospital that have to be taken into account.

- The first is as a place of healing, which emphasizes throughput, like a factory, and is closest to the managerial model.

- The second is as a place of caring, where the emphasis is on the process, which may be long-term or even permanent. Questions that tend to arise here are about loss and grief, hope and meaning. This is the nursing or hospice model.

- Third is the educational purpose, training people into the healing, caring arts and skills, and openly visible in the teaching hospital.

- Last, comes the 'living, learning arena model':

    Because the imports and exports are human beings we (and our families) are responding to events, experiencing from them, learning from them... The hospital is a school for society in which attitudes to illness and health, ageing and death are taught. (Wilson 1971, pp.2–3)

Perhaps it is the chaplain's task to start at this end and to be a catalyst in this wider, integrative and fundamental responsibility and perspective. However, this is a role that is increasingly difficult to sustain in the contemporary setting.

Chaplains as professionals

The dilemmas that chaplains are now experiencing are illustrated by the issue of professionalism. The Health Professions Council has been trying, as part of its task, to come up with a definition of a modern health care profession, integral to the so-called programme of 'modernization', which questions the notion of professional monopoly and power by blurring the boundaries between them and strengthening the accountability structures:

The Council proposes that any 'occupational group' eligible for regulation will be required to demonstrate the following features:

- They cover a discrete area of activity (not all of which need be exclusively theirs) displaying some homogeneity.

- They apply a defined body of knowledge and practice based on evidence of efficacy. A good test of efficacy will be acceptability to the medical profession [sic!].

- They have an established professional body (which accounts for a significant proportion of that group).

- The professional body also operates a voluntary register of entry to the profession and entry qualification that are independently assessed.

- They operate a defined code of practice and ethical standards with disciplinary procedures.

- They are of a size that makes registration a practical and cost effective proposition.

(Health Professions Council 2002, p.140)

Hospital chaplains, as evidenced by this and the previous discussion, are in a cleft stick. Do they strengthen and secure their position by seeking recognition among the accepted health professional groups and fight their corner from within? Or do they remain on the fringe, relying on the continuing good will of the NHS management, both locally and nationally?

Moreover, there is another difficulty. The professional structures of the churches are notoriously weak and are not obviously health care orientated. Also there has been growing unease with the way the churches currently undervalue sector (non-parochial) ministries, raising the spectre of insecurity from that quarter as well (Swift 2005). But for the chaplains to set up even a semi-independent organization threatens traditional ecclesiastical authority. In addition nowadays the presence of other religious groups has also to be taken into account, adding further confusion to an already opaque situation.

The tendency, although there remains a wide spectrum of opinions on this, has been to move towards greater professionalization in order to try to secure an accepted place in the health service. This has led to the formation of the College of Health Care Chaplains (CHCC) in England and Wales, alongside the Association of Hospice and Palliative Care Chaplains and the Scottish Association of Chaplains in Health Care. Another step in this journey was the affiliation of the College, as an autonomous section, to the trades union Unite (Swift 2006).

Perhaps the greatest difficulties that face the chaplains in their desire to be accepted as a profession are the two core criteria of a defined body of knowledge and practice and evidence of efficacy, especially when measured against the core medical professions. The expected pattern is of a body of knowledge that is mastered and applied through learned skills. Sometimes it is assumed (mistakenly) that a faith tradition works this way – providing answers to given issues out of an authorized tradition. But, in fact, the chaplain works out of a tradition of 'practical wisdom', which provides a context for reflective appraisal in seeking an appropriate response. The focus is on the person in their particularity. It is, therefore, essentially a dialogue in which the *client* determines the direction and outcome. This puts the chaplain closer to mentor and friend than professional expert. Such wisdom is not encapsulated in a body of knowledge and practice in the same way as, say, engineering. Christian theology is essentially a form of participative discourse – a notoriously diffuse and permeable subject area. Other faith traditions also have their own ways of handing down and developing their traditions. Moreover and importantly, such wisdom cannot be separated from the person of the chaplain. There is a relationship between the practitioner and the practice that entails a certain kind of personal commitment, often called 'vocation'.

Such a sense of 'calling' is not uncommon among those who seek 'to work with people', and has been traditionally very much part of the caring and medical professions; but it is a model that has been widely neglected and even discounted in the 'modernized' professional context. Clearly for the clergy this remains significant. Yet, questions of motivation and the relevance of personal qualities will still remain for others in the health care professions, even for those who may not accept a metaphysical perspective. It is argued that a strong sense of dedication and service is still important. It would be tragic if all perception of vocation were to disappear. Perhaps it is part of the chaplains' task to ensure that such a discourse is sustained (Ballard 2004, pp.47–55).

It is also almost impossible to measure pastoral effectiveness (Mowat 2008). There is clear evidence that the chaplaincy service is widely appreciated. There are, too, studies that suggest that the religious dimension has a positive correlation with better health rates (Wright 2005). Chaplains are also often welcome at points of crisis when they can bring resources and handle dimensions that are not always possible for hard-pressed medical teams to meet. But all this is hard to quantify (Orchard 2000, pp.120–122). Swift characterizes this as being a 'friend', so that chaplains are valued 'not for technical ability but for personal care and mindfulness' (Swift 2004, p.11). How can these elements be regarded as a professional task under the conditions imposed today?

Nevertheless, somewhat cautiously, the key chaplaincy organizations are inching towards trying to find professional acceptability under the HPC or similar body. The College of Health Care Chaplains, with the churches' relevant authorities, has produced a set of professional standards or competencies (over the period 1993–1998). These outline the expected skills and training required. The three UK associations for health care chaplains (Association of Hospice and Palliative Care Chaplains; Scottish Association of Chaplains in Health Care; College of Health Care Chaplains) have worked on a Code of Conduct, which they describe as 'a major step forward in the development of the profession and provides a basis for greater confidence in the care we give' (2005, p.2). They have also set up a Chaplaincy Academic and Accreditation Board that, using the Standards for the Chaplaincy Service of NHS Scotland (NHS Scotland 2007; also see Scottish Executive Health Department 2002), gives recognition to the small but increasing number of courses available, such as the induction course at HE level 2 (Cardiff), and masters degrees in Leeds (Health Care Chaplaincy) and Cardiff (Chaplaincy, with a health care pathway). It is also recognized that, to meet 'evidence based' criteria now governing the NHS, there is a need for well-focused and targeted research (Mowat 2008). Furthermore, there is currently emerging a new body called the UK Board of Health Care Chaplaincy to represent the interests of each of the professional membership bodies.

WORKING IN A MULTI-FAITH SOCIETY

Over past decades British society has consciously recognized its pluralistic and multi-faith nature. As a result, religion has taken on a much higher profile in public affairs. This has also had the effect of radically changing the religious landscape from one of Christian establishment (dominated by Anglicanism) to a more diverse pattern, and has been a challenge to the widely assumed secularization of Western culture. It is now, therefore, increasingly assumed that non-Christian faiths will provide (as the Jews long have) spiritual and religious support for their adherents within the public structures such as the NHS. In some Trusts, where demand warrants it, this now includes the appointment of chaplains, usually part-time, from other faiths, predominantly Islam. This has had interesting repercussions.

At one level the NHS can provide what seems a straightforward solution. Committed to enabling all patients to have spiritual and religious care, the new religious communities simply slot into the provision as agreed with the Multi-faith Group for Hospital Chaplaincy and currently set out in *NHS Chaplaincy: Meeting the Religious and Spiritual Needs of Patients and Staff* (Multi-faith Group for Health Care Chaplaincy 2003). There are, however, a number of acute issues that have to be faced and that will probably only get resolved over time, but which could, meanwhile, produce controversy.

First, there is the problem of which groupings should be included. There is little dispute over the larger and more established faiths; but, in an increasingly fragmented society in which personal preference is paramount, smaller groups will also be pressing for recognition. This can include new and sometimes somewhat bizarre faiths; and what about groups on the Christian fringe such as Mormons and Christian Science? All religions are themselves fragmented and have their own internal variations reflecting historical, cultural, racial and theological (sometimes acute) differences.

There is then the practical problem of religious principles and practice in the hospital situation that may well clash with medical procedures and norms. This has, of course, been recognized to some extent already, such as Catholic objections to abortion or Jehovah's Witnesses to blood transfusion, or the way in which death and the disposal of the body is dealt with among Sikhs, Muslims or Jews. Clearly it is possible to provide guidelines and directives for the medical and nursing staff. However, this is potentially a minefield of ethical and cultural issues for which it would be impossible to prepare every member of staff for every contingency. This may well be one of the important tasks of the chaplaincy team: interpreting and mediating between the medical world and the members of different faith groups.

Behind this there is an underlying problem that there is currently no agreement as to what it means to be a multi-cultural society. A society in flux and increasingly diverse can lose its cohesion, threatening instability and conflict. It is also true that the relation of an immigrant group with the host culture changes with time and the economic context. At present the government wavers between some form of inclusivity and encouraging diversity. Perhaps these are not mutually exclusive aims and over a number of generations, a new national identity will inevitably emerge, drawing on and modifying these different traditions including religion (which is always responding to the changing society around).

At present, however, the common nomenclature is of 'faith communities'. It is not clear whether this primarily refers to fairly distinct, perhaps ethnically based religious groupings or is a generic term for any religious voluntary activity. This ambiguity is to be found in the way Christian churches are often, in practice, not given the recognition of 'faith communities' in the same way as mosques or gurdwaras. This perhaps reflects the historic cultural status of Christianity in Britain, in which, today, C of E is one set of traditions alongside others in a secular context.

Spirituality in the health care setting

There has been, however, another unexpected development that seems to give support to the chaplains' cause. The rising interest in 'spirituality' across society has got onto the health care agenda, producing a concern for 'holistic' care, which 'may be defined as the integration of the physical, social, psychological and spiritual aspects of the person' (Cobb and Robshaw 1998, p.2). Having long been at the root of much hospice care (Murray 2002), this has now entered into the curriculum in a significant way in nursing. There is now a significant and growing research literature on the subject and relevant diagnostic and caring practices are now being developed (Kliewer and Saultz 2006; Whipp 2001).

Spirituality is, of course, a slippery concept, described by Pattison as functioning 'like intellectual polyfilla, changing shape and content conveniently to fill the space its users devise for it' (Pattison 2001, p.37). The impetus, however, has been towards an inclusive, generic use of the term. It has almost, where it has been taken up, become a technical term for that existential sense of meaning that is assumed to be at the core of our experience, which may or may not be strongly articulated, or even acknowledged. It varies from person to person. It may or may not be coherent, or flexible. It can be creative but also destructive. It may or may not be expressed through religious faith and practice. Indeed, spirituality and religion are often contrasted because the former is seen as being inward and personal and as wider and comprehensive (which is assumed to be 'a good thing') and the latter as more external, authoritative, divisive and limiting ('a bad thing'). Victor Frankl, who has become something of a guru, argues that human beings are essentially 'meaning creating' creatures (White 2006, 97ff), while others appeal to the way Paul Tournier, the Swiss doctor-theologian, intergrates faith perspectives and healing (Cox, Campbell and Fulford 2007).

This trend however, interestingly, introduces a counter-culture into the medical process itself. Spirituality stresses the individuality of the patient. There cannot be a prescriptive approach (though there are some who would wish to work along these lines, translating spirituality into quantifiable elements (Cobb 1998)). Here is the ultimate in consumer choice. This view is much closer to counselling of a non-directive kind, which engages with the client/patient in a process of reflective self-awareness in order to understand their own dynamics, on the basis of which they can learn the better to cope with the traumas of illness. The health professional thus becomes a catalyst opening up possibilities for change and growth rather than an analyst and prescriber of treatment:

> Such a change of approach recognizes the importance of building patient autonomy and requires health professionals to work differently, developing new communication and other skills such as listening and building relationships. (White 2006, p.37)

It is also axiomatic that to do this the counsellor is also engaged at a personal and emotional level and needs to have considerable self-awareness and skills in dealing with 'transference' and 'counter-transference'.[1] So White, when discussing the training process for nurses and others, suggests:

> Simply presenting information about spirituality is unlikely to engage participants in any personal exploration; a reflective educational approach encourages participants to learn more deeply as they consider spirituality in the light of their own personal and professional experience. (White 2006, p.45)

Thus introducing spirituality as an element in nursing and other areas of health care is making a tall order on professionals who need to be expert and busy in other areas of medicine. It also has interesting repercussions for the recruitment process and a sense of vocation.

Whether spiritual care is a task proper to nursing or any of the others on the medical team is a discussion that must be conducted elsewhere (Bradshaw 1994; Clarke 2004). For the chaplains, however, it is an important recent development. On one hand, it challenges what has hitherto looked like their monopoly, while, on the other, it draws their traditional concern into the mainstream of medical practice. If spirituality as an aspect of patient care were to be accepted then the chaplains' theological training and professional formation would carry much greater credibility, for these are exactly the issues that will have been worked on there. However, this is a variant on the dilemma posed by religious pluralism, i.e. what does it mean to be a chaplain, with a clear faith mandate, to work in this open-ended way? There is some evidence that what the patients at least look for is what could be called 'open integrity'. That is, they want the chaplain to be what he or she is, a priest of the Church. That is their identity. But they also want a person who is open and welcoming, who accepts people as they are, with no strings attached. Nurses have their own tasks, to care but not to counsel. The chaplain is there precisely to attend to those areas that the medical staff are not there primarily to address, such as meaning, anxiety, hopes, relationships, reconnecting to discarded roots or reaching out to a greater reality, which is perhaps God (Ballard *et al.* 1999, 2000) So,

---

1   Transference, used in a psychological sense, is 'the redirection of emotions originally felt in childhood' on to another person, so that it distorts an inter-personal relationship. Counter-transference describes the way the emotional reaction of the therapist or counsellor to the patient can impede objectivity or clarity in the therapeutic relationship.

there are gains and losses for the chaplains. David Lyall (2001) indicates this thus:

> [Spirituality] is a celebration of the human spirit and here we have its strength and limitation. Its strength lies in its vision of the person as more than a machine; its limitation, from a Christian perspective, is that God becomes at best an optional extra, one particular expression of the transcendent. (p.49)

What lies ahead?

There would appear, therefore, to be a number of options currently facing chaplaincy teams and individual chaplains.

- It is, of course, possible for chaplains to minister only to those of their own faith. To act in this way, however, would tend to weaken any ties with, and commitment to, the wider health institution.

- Chaplaincy teams can try to diversify to cover all the bases; but, compounded by limited resources, this is going to prove impossible beyond token levels. Moreover, different faiths have very different understandings of pastoral care. The Christian Priest, the Jewish rabbi and the Muslim imam, for example, relate to their people and their tasks in surprisingly different ways. It is hard to see how realistically such diversity can be integrated into a really cohesive team. Where such teams do work there is also reason to suggest that it depends on the coming together of a very particular group of people who may not be totally representative of their several faiths. In another situation there could be a completely different mix.

- It is possible for each chaplain to try to offer a ministry in an open way beyond their own faith community. This can be supplemented by having a group of specialists on call to respond to particular demands. This, too, is open to the limitations of local resources and a possible open-ended demand. At the same time there are many who would be suspicious of, or reject, the ministrations from those not of their faith community.

- The fourth approach tries to subvert the problem by seeking some kind of generic solution, on the assumption that there is a common basic spirituality that underlies all faiths and that it is possible to work at this level, though recognizing that this reality is expressed in myriad ways (whether expressed religiously or through some humanistic philosophy or in other form). This is clearly attractive to the administrator, chiming in with the modernist principle of looking for the universal behind the diversity, and thus would make it easier to integrate the spiritual dimension into the medical provision. The chaplain thereby makes the claim to offer this expertise within the care team, complementing the medical, nursing and welfare staff.

Chaplains appear to waver between these various possibilities according to conviction, need and opportunity. Because they are charged within the health service with a potentially universal task there is a clear tension between that and their denominational or other allegiances. This is parallel to the priest in an Anglican parish, who is expected to relate not only to the active congregation but also to the community at large. There is no simple answer. All that can be expected is to be flexible, honest, open and willing to straddle roles.

It is also interesting to note here that it is not unusual for the senior chaplain to be on the Trust's Ethical Committee. Here the same tension holds. On the one hand, they are the source of information about religious beliefs and moral values, themselves assumed to have a moral standpoint. On the other hand, they also have relevant skills, training and experience, not least in ethical discourse, that can assist in arriving at a common mind in the face of some of the many ethical dilemmas posed by modern medicine that impinge even at the local level. To carry out this role, however, there has to be a high degree of openness on the part of the chaplain to the perspectives and values that inform medical science and research and society as a whole.

CONCLUSIONS

This chapter has tried to set out some of the key tensions and threats facing health care chaplains in a changing NHS in a changing society. To some extent they are having to defend their legitimate place in the health care system, where they are exposed to cuts, even though it can be argued that the service is cheap at the price (Grote 2007). However, there is an irony here. Just at the point when chaplains are agonizing over how to defend their role as 'clown' or guardians of the 'soul' (in Foucault's sense of a disembodied or non-corporeal locus of behaviour (Swift 2004)), from the midst of the health service comes the desire to address issues of 'spirit' and meaning, which suggests that there is a place for something akin to chaplaincy, however it may modify itself in the future.

Given all this agonizing, what is actually happening on the ground? There are about 300 full-time, and hundreds more part-time, chaplains, as well as volunteers, actually moving around our hospitals daily. But Orchard (2000), surveying the chaplaincy service in London, found great variation both in approach and in how chaplaincy was understood, both in the hospital and in the chaplaincy team. Teams were sometimes very much on the margins, there under sufferance; but elsewhere were seen as a core part of the Trust's provision. There were also signs of adapting to new patterns of health provision and some moving out into the community. Nor was acceptability or effectiveness dependent on the theological or theoretical models of pastoral care adopted. Traditional ways of working appeared to be no better or worse than an open-ended 'spirituality'. Similarly there is no set template for multi-faith chaplaincy teams. Nor is there any consistency about how the hospital chaplains team relates to the local or wider 'faith communities'. Perhaps the last word can come from Helen Orchard (2000):

> One of the very real challenges in today's NHS is balancing the desire to care for people in a humane and holistic way with the need to deliver that care in an efficiently mechanistic manner. The NHS needs help in not losing sight of the people it is serving while it improves the process of serving them... Chaplains, if they chose to, have every opportunity to make a significant contribution to the achievement of that goal, which is to be delivered within a culture of equality, reliability, accountability and, of course, compassion. (p.152)

RESPONSE
Chris Swift

Paul Ballard's well-observed and effective analysis of the chaplain sets out what are the principal challenges for the profession. For chaplains, the debate has not moved far from primary questions, including, 'Can chaplaincy be meaningfully spoken of as a profession'? For some, chaplains are simply an expression of a church or faith community: hence they possess no collegial or corporate identity across religious divides. For others, chaplaincy has become a new multi-faith entity, pivoting on the common focus of the patient, and united by a shared experience of working in the NHS. These differences of approach have intensified in recent years, with greater faith-specific guidance (e.g. Catholic Bishops' Conference of England and Wales, Department for Christian Responsibility and Citizenship, Health Care Reference Group 2007) emerging alongside new non-denominational structures such as the UK Board of Health Care Chaplaincy. At times it can feel that, if there is a balance in chaplaincy, it is the kind found between people sitting at opposite ends of the same see-saw.

In what follows I want briefly to respond to two issues in Paul Ballard's piece: secularization and vocation.

SECULARIZATION

It is Tuesday and a patient has just died on one of the wards. He was a local taxi driver. His wife – from a nominally Christian upbringing – knows that despite a total lack of practice during their married life her husband wished to be buried as a Muslim. She has no idea how to arrange this. The Muslim and Christian chaplains are invited to be involved, supporting and facilitating the honouring of his last wish. The man's wife expects to be present at the burial – but this is not normal Islamic practice in this part of West Yorkshire. Something is arranged, a place to stand and watch. Everything is moving ahead smoothly and swiftly. Then the man's brother arrives from London. 'No,' he says, 'in the part of Africa we come from Muslims are buried on a Friday.' Despite the surprise this gives the Muslim chaplain, used to the general rule of burial as soon as possible, the arrangements are amended and the wishes of all concerned are, eventually, respected.

Good chaplaincy works across boundaries. The next-of-kin in the above scenario falls into that great category of British people who identify with Christianity but have chosen not to participate in Church life. It is matched by the emerging phenomenon in the West of those from other faiths who equally lack direct involvement with the structures of their faith. The actions of the chaplains are not about claiming individuals for their particular cause, but about supporting and respecting the wishes of all concerned: deceased; widow; brother. To quote Paul Ballard, this is an example of 'open integrity', where chaplains draw on their skill and knowledge to meet the unique needs of each situation. No one expects chaplains to disown their convictions in the face of human suffering and sorrow, but they *are* expected to work together to achieve an outcome capable of sustaining meaning for all the parties involved. For some observers this shift away from signed-up religious belonging is evidence of a secularization creeping through every sector of society – including the NHS. Both the deceased patient and his widow show elements of religious formation (or, at least, linkage) but one wonders whether this would apply to the generation after them.

Paul Ballard's analysis touches on this tension between the chaplain's faith-specific identity and the population's declining orthodoxy and growing diversity. However, while the traditional practice of Christianity in Europe is a shadow of its former self, there appears to be little appetite for a thorough-going embrace of atheism. More often than not chaplains encounter those who hold and cherish fragments of the Christian faith, but who are unwilling to surrender the definition of their faith to figures of religious authority. During research between 2000 and 2001 the hesitancy about formal belief in the patients I visited was a recurring theme.

VOCATION

As a chaplain I recognize the threats and opportunities Ballard identifies for the chaplain in the shifting arena of modern health care. The twentieth century marked a removal of religious matters from the centre to the margin, and this is well illustrated by the fact that the size and splendour of Victorian hospital chapels has been replaced by smaller, informal and more abstract places of contemplation variously called 'the sanctuary', 'quiet room' or 'multi-faith space'. As the declarative function of religion in the public square has been questioned and squeezed out, hospital chapels offer a fascinating testimony of social change. From the creation of buildings little different from parish churches there came the 'friendlier' chapels of the 1960s with soft furnishings and ambient lighting, to be followed at the close of the Millennium by plain rooms inspired (if at all) by modern art installations and natural wood finishes. Once you were told; now you must surmise.

Running parallel to these physical changes there is, possibly, a less obvious, and more debatable, transformation of the chaplain's inner convictions. The leading writers about chaplaincy in the mid-twentieth century (Autton 1966; Cox 1955; Wilson 1971) held a high view of the chaplain's vocation to care for the sick and to support NHS staff. In effect, these writers drew on widely accepted assumptions about the idea of 'calling' and how it was vocation that led certain priests into work within the NHS. While no historical study of factors leading clergy into the NHS has been undertaken, there is plenty of anecdotal evidence to suggest that it sometimes in fact had more to do with getting someone out of a parish than getting them into a hospital! Research into contemporary Anglican hospital chaplains showed this starkly when it revealed that over 20 per cent of male chaplains in its sample stated that they were in a same-sex relationship (Hancocks, Sherbourne and Swift 2008).

The trouble with 'vocation' is that it has been a term widely abused in many different ways. For women it was used as a way to dignify the intimacies of nursing while allowing pay to be suppressed in comparison with male occupations. Remarkably, this debate still continues in some quarters (Heyes 2005). If vocation is to be meaningfully rehabilitated there must be greater openness and honesty about the factors leading people to work as either nurses or chaplains. It is still a valuable term, if only because it suggests – akin to 'spirituality' – that contractual material arrangements are not wholly satisfactory. Pay should be fair, but there are also ethical commitments to those in the care of the professional, and these should be honoured whenever humanly possible. At its best, vocation is about being who we are more fully because we answer a sense of inner or outer calling. In the NHS the context for vocation is among patients often facing episodes of crisis and change in their lives. We owe it to these patients to take the idea of vocation seriously – and not use it as a disguise to excuse poor pay or hide those clergy whose personal integrity raises too many inconvenient questions.

CONCLUSIONS

In a Western world living through unprecedented social change it seems unthinkable that the NHS could abandon the skills of those uniquely placed to link the past to the present. Although eager atheists are keen to see the NHS dispense with its chaplains (and are unwittingly attacking a group of clerics often at odds with religious orthodoxy), it would be a mistake to think that the hard-wiring of spirituality into Western living is so easily suspended: 'the time that was continues to tick inside the time that is' (Berger 2008, p.85). While they teeter between their historic origins and the possibilities of greater professional coherence, the position of chaplains embodies a wider disquiet with both religious authority and secular stridency. It is not clear at present whether chaplains possess the determination, the capacity or the desire to learn from their uniquely public dilemma. But, I believe, such an engagement is to be encouraged because there are plenty of reasons to believe that their self-understanding can have wider relevance for other professions.

REFERENCES

Association of Hospice and Palliative Care Chaplains, Scottish Association of Chaplains in Health Care, College of Health Care Chaplains (2005) *Health Care Chaplains – Code of Conduct* (2nd edn). Assocn. of Hospice and Palliative Care Chaplains, Scottish Assn. of Chaplains in Health Care, College of Health Care Chaplains.

Autton, N. (1966) *The Hospital Ministry*. London: Church Information Office.

Ballard, P. (2004) 'The Clergy: An Interesting Anomaly.' In S. Pattison and R. Pill (eds) (2004) *Values in Professional Practice – Lessons for Health, Social Care and other Professionals*. Oxford: Radcliffe.

Ballard, P., Finlay, I., Roberts, S., Searle, C. and Jones, N. (1999) 'A perception of hospital chaplaincy.' *Contact 130*, 24–34.

Ballard, P., Finlay, I., Jones, N., Searle, C. and Roberts, S. (2000) 'Spiritual perspectives among terminally ill patients – a Welsh sample.' *Modern Believing 41*, 2, 30–38.

Berger, J. (2008) *From A to X*. London: Verso.

Bradshaw, A. (1994) *Lighting the Lamp – The Spiritual Dimension of Nursing Care*. Harrow: Scutari.

Catholic Bishops' Conference of England and Wales, Department for Christian Responsibility and Citizenship, Health Care Reference Group (2007) *Caring for the Catholic Patient: Meeting the Pastoral Needs of Catholic Patients*. London: Catholic Truth Society.

Clarke, J. (2004) *Nursing and Spirituality – a Theological Approach*. Cardiff University: PhD thesis.

Cobb, M. (1998) 'Assessing Spiritual Need – An Examination in Practice.' In M. Cobb and V. Robshaw (eds) *The Spiritual Challenge of Health Care*. London: Churchill Livingstone.

Cobb, M. and Robshaw, V. (1998) *The Spiritual Challenge of Health Care*. London: Churchill Livingstone.

Cox, J. (1955) *A Priest's Work in Hospital*. London: Society for Promoting Christian Knowledge.

Cox, J., Campbell, A.V. and Fulford, B. (eds) (2007) *Medicine of the Person – Faith, Science and Values in Health Care Provision*. London: Jessica Kingsley Publishers.

Faber, H. (1971) *Pastoral Care in a Modern Hospital*. London: Student Christian Movement.

Grote, D. (2007) 'Hospital chaplains axed to cut costs, says report.' *Baptist Times*, 11 October 2007.

Hancocks, G.J., Sherbourne, B. and Swift, C. (2008) 'Are they refugees? Why Church of England clergy enter health care chaplaincy.' *Practical Theology 1*, 2, 163–179.

Health Professions Council (2002) *The Future (A Paper for Consultation)*. London: Health Professions Council.

Heyes, A. (2005) 'The economics of vocation or "why is a badly paid nurse a good nurse"?' *Journal of Health Economics 24*, 3, 561–569.

Hospital Chaplains' Council (1978) *A Handbook on Hospital Chaplaincy*. London: Church Information Office.

Kliewer, S.P. and Saultz, J. (2006) *Health Care and Spirituality*. Oxford: Radcliffe.

Lambourne, B. (1983) 'Towards an Understanding of Medico-Theological Dialogue.' In M. Wilson (ed.) *Explorations in Health and Salvation – a Selection of Papers by Bob Lambourne*. Birmingham: University of Birmingham Institute for the Study of Worship and Religious Architecture.

Lyall, D. (2001) *The Integrity of Pastoral Care*. London: Society for Promoting Christian Knowledge.

McSherry, W. (2006) *Making Sense of Spirituality in Nursing and Health Care Practice*. London: Jessica Kingsley Publishers.

Mowat, H. (2008) *The Potential for Efficacy of Health Care Chaplaincy and Spiritual Care Provision in the NHS (UK): A Scoping Review of Recent Research*. NHS: Yorkshire and the Humber.

Multi-faith Group for Health Care Chaplaincy (2003) *NHS Chaplaincy – Meeting the Religious and Spiritual Needs of Patients and Staff. Guidance for Managers and Those Involved in the Provision of Chaplaincy-Spiritual Care*. London: Multi-faith Group for Health Care Chaplaincy.

Murray, D. (2002) *Faith in Hospices – Spiritual Care and the End of Life*. London: Society for Promoting Christian Knowledge.

NHS Scotland (2007) *Standards for the Chaplaincy Service*. Edinburgh: NHS Scotland.

Orchard, H. (2000) *Hospital Chaplaincy – Modern, Dependable?* Lincoln Theological Institute Research Project, 1. Sheffield: Sheffield Academic Press.

Orchard, H. (ed.) (2001) *Spirituality in Health Care Contexts*. London: Jessica Kingsley Publishers.

Pattison, S. (1997) *The Faith of the Managers*. London: Cassell.

Pattison, S. (2001) 'Dumbing Down the Spirit.' In H. Orchard (ed.) *Spirituality in Health Care Contexts*. London: Jessica Kingsley Publishers.

Scottish Executive Health Department (2002) *Guidelines on Chaplaincy and Spiritual Care in the NHS Scotland*. Edinburgh: NHS Scotland: NHS HDL 76.

South Yorkshire Strategic Health Authority (2003) *Caring for the Spirit – A Strategy for the Chaplaincy and Spiritual Health Care Workforce*. Sheffield: South Yorkshire Strategic Health Authority.

Swift, C. (2004) 'How should health care chaplaincy negotiate its professional identity?' *Contact 144*, 4–13.

Swift, C. (2005) *The Function of the Chaplain in the Government of the Sick in English Acute Hospitals*. Sheffield University: PhD thesis.

Swift, C. (2006) 'Political awakening of contemporary chaplaincy.' *The Journal of Health Care Chaplains 7*, 1, 57–62.

Whipp, M. (2001) 'Discerning the Spirits: Theological Audit in Health Care Organizations.' In H. Orchard (ed.) *Spirituality in Health Care Contexts*. London: Jessica Kingsley Publishers.

White, G. (2006) *Talking about Spirituality in Health Care Practice – A Resource for the Multi-professional Health Care Team*. London: Jessica Kingsley Publishers.

Wilson, M. (1971) *The Hospital – A Place of Truth*. Birmingham: University of Birmingham Institute for the Study of Worship and Religious Architecture.

Wright, S.G. (2005) *Reflections on Spirituality and Health*. London: Whurr.

Chapter 10

What Are the Values of NHS Managers, and How Have they Changed since 1983?

Stephen Pattison and Julia McKeown

INTRODUCTION

A popular stereotype of National Health Service (NHS) managers represented in TV soap operas and reflected in some existing literature is that of the uncommitted, ruthless 'suit' whose focus is on the 'bottom line' of expenditure and on meeting business targets instead of upon the concerns of clinical staff for patients and services (see Draper 1998). Managers in the NHS are often regarded as the vectors of undesirable values and change by both the public and other health care professions. It is, therefore, important to establish what values they actually espouse and enact, and whether these have changed since formal management was introduced into the NHS in 1983. Our approach here has been informed by reviewing existing research literature and by undertaking discussions with current NHS managers.

WHAT IS AN NHS MANAGER?

Problems in understanding the past and present values of managers arise as soon as one starts trying to identify what a contemporary NHS manager might be. A manager is likely to be, but not necessarily, an NHS employee. The term 'manager' can include a number of disparate roles – from clinicians who undertake the administrative direction of a service, to managers undertaking generic organizational functions such as finance or human resources, to executive managers forming part of the top-tier governance of an organization. Management experiences and values may be affected by seniority within the organization; and managers undertake their roles at different levels, from wards to Trusts. Furthermore, these functions may take place within widely different organizational settings, e.g. Primary Care Trusts, Foundation or Acute NHS Trusts, Mental Health Trusts, and Care Trusts.

What do managers do, and what are the values of management?

Essentially managers deliver. They do things. They make it happen. In other words, they are pragmatic functionaries. Modern managers are basically the product of twentieth-century, mostly commercial, industrial organization (Drucker 1974; Locke 1996). Indeed, many managers have no professional background at all; and there is often no necessity to have any formal qualifications or training to manage. The main attribute needed is a willingness and ability to get work done through and with other people (Pattison 1997).

Managers have a job to do. This is essentially to direct flows of resources 'to achieve defined objectives' (Pollitt 1993, p.5). Their prime purpose is 'to do what they are best at – getting things done' (Wall 2004, p.74). They pursue calculated definite ends with a clear intention of bringing about successful outcomes (Hewison 2002).

Within this utilitarian, calculating, pragmatic horizon, managers aim to improve organizational performance by:

- setting objectives

- organizing activities, relations and decisions

- integrating activity by communication and motivation

- measuring individual and corporate performance against pre-set targets

- developing and improving people, including themselves (see Drucker 1974, pp.20–21).

Once the tasks of management as forecasting and planning, organizing, coordinating, commanding and controlling have been identified (see Pugh and Hickson 1989, p.86), perhaps one has said all that can usefully be said about the values of NHS managers. This may not be a particularly exalted or philosophically complex role, but it is a necessary one.

Managers in the NHS

While management may be a necessary function, the NHS survived formally without it for its first 35 years. It was only in 1983 that a Conservative government, as part of a wholesale review of the perceived inadequacies, costliness and inefficiency of state-provided services, asked Sir Roy Griffiths to make recommendations about NHS organization (DHSS 1983). Before Griffiths, the NHS was professionally led, but supported by an administrative function designed to facilitate clinical activity (Strong and Robinson 1990). Administrators essentially follow laid-down rules and principles and tend to be concerned with processes, activities and keeping things going (du Gay 2005). However, administered organizations tend to over-supply services and to maximize budget expenditure. Griffiths recommended the immediate implementation of general management at all levels in order to produce radical cultural change.

It is perhaps in Griffiths' brief report that the foundational values of contemporary NHS management are to be found. Cox (1992) notes:

> The recurring themes [of Griffiths] are 'management action', 'effectiveness', 'accountability', 'performance', 'decision-making', 'driving force', 'responsibility', 'devolution', 'leadership', 'initiative, urgency and vitality', 'thrust, commitment and energy', and 'new style'. (p.5)

The values of NHS managers

It might be thought that under the influence of Griffiths and other practices and ideas derived from the private sector that NHS managers would value most, if not all the following, in a fairly unadulterated way:

- effectiveness
- efficiency
- economy

- accountability
- competition
- multiplicity of providers
- scepticism about state-provided services and professional protectionism and monopolies
- consumer orientation and choice
- entrepreneurialism and innovation
- flexibility and responsiveness
- clear decision-making and line responsibilities
- target setting
- measurement and control
- outcomes over processes
- constant improvement
- organizational over individual good and interests
- obedience to organizational superiors and politicians.

However, private sector values have not necessarily materialized in practice. Within the complex context of the NHS, managers have to take account of professional values, bureaucratic values, local values and priorities, and the political values of the public sector (Clarke, Cochrane and McLaughlin 1994; du Gay 2005; Ranson and Stewart 1994). The managers have adapted in the context of the service and the localities in which they work to become an integral part of the NHS.

Managers are primarily doers, not thinkers or theorists. They do not spend much time formally articulating or analyzing values, but their work is not value-free and they do have values and concerns. However, the few formal statements of NHS management values that exist are not very informative.

The 2001 Institute of Health care Management (IHM) Code of Conduct requires members to:

- exhibit integrity (do not pursue own interests or accept gifts and favours, safeguard confidential information)
- exhibit honesty and openness

- exhibit probity (use resources responsibly and efficiently)
- exhibit accountability (justify actions under political scrutiny)
- exhibit respect (for colleagues, employees, patients)
- exhibit respect for the environment (health and safety)
- exhibit respect and understanding for society and community
- engage in professional development.

IHM has a membership of less than 10 per cent of all NHS managers, so this code, while uncontroversial and useful as an iteration of basic values, is not binding on all managers (Wall 2004). The Department of Health's Code of Conduct (2002) is, however, an authoritative document. This requires managers to adhere to the following standards, against which they can be disciplined:

- respect patient confidentiality
- use resources in an effective, efficient and timely manner in the best interests of the public and patients
- ensure a safe working environment
- protect patients from risk
- treat anyone with concerns reasonably and fairly
- respect and treat with dignity and fairness the public, patients, relatives, carers, NHS staff and partners in other agencies
- ensure no one is unlawfully discriminated against
- be honest and act with probity and integrity
- accept responsibility for their own work and the performance of people managed
- be accountable to the public, patients, relatives, carers, NHS staff, partners
- be committed to teamwork
- take responsibility for own learning and development.

Both these documents show clear influence from the principles of public life identified by the Nolan Committee in 1995, which are: selflessness (public interest); integrity (not being influenced from outside); objectivity (making choices on merit); accountability (openness to scrutiny); openness (about decisions and actions); honesty (about conflicts of interest); leadership (supporting these principles) (see Lawton 1998, p.46). The Nolan principles reflect the unwritten components of the so-called 'public service ethic' which comprises 'honesty, integrity, impartiality, recruitment and promotion on merit, probity, accountability...' (Lawton 1998, p.51). All of which perhaps suggests that it is very difficult within the public sector to develop unfettered, red-blooded managerial entrepreneurialism without having to take account of traditional bureaucratic and political values within a complex context (du Gay 2005).

This reference to documents reveals little about how NHS managers actually adopt, interpret and enact values on the ground, nor how they interact with the values of the NHS organizations and health care professions with which they have to work on an everyday basis. What, then, is known of NHS managers' values in practice?

STUDYING THE VALUES OF NHS MANAGERS

It is difficult to talk authoritatively about the operant espoused and enacted values of NHS managers as a group in practice for a variety of reasons. First, very few studies of public sector managers' values have been undertaken. Second, as already noted, health services managers are not a homogeneous group in terms of background, socialization, context, level or experience.

Furthermore, many managers actually come from clinical backgrounds and are steeped in the practical care of individuals and a professional ethos of providing the best care possible for those individuals. These 'hybrid' managers (Ferlie et al. 1996; Hewison 2002) bring with them a concern for the welfare of individuals and on-the-ground care delivery that dilutes any simple adoption of Taylorist values that might be implicit in the origins of management in the world of private enterprise.

The study of NHS management values is a complex and multi-layered activity and very few studies have been undertaken in this area. There are very few useful autobiographical accounts of managers' lives in the NHS from which operant values might be deduced (but see Edwards 1993). Those that do exist mostly do not deal directly with the values of the individuals concerned. Here, however, is a summary of some of the studies that might be relevant.

Lawton (1998) and others undertook a small-scale questionnaire of 45 public sector managers (level of responsibility and organization worked in not disclosed) undertaking the MBA at the Open University. They asked what managers thought the operant and the desirable principles were that should pertain in public sector management. The top operant principles identified were meeting targets, obeying rules, obeying superiors, political awareness and competitiveness, while many of the formally approved public-sector management values of leadership, objectivity, loyalty, thoroughness, selflessness and exercising initiative were at the bottom of the list. These managers thought that integrity, accountability, responding to the client/customer, openness and commitment to a public service ethos should be the key desirable principles or values for managing public services and that obeying rules and superiors should be right at the bottom of the normative list (Lawton 1998, p.47)!

Summarizing a number of studies of public sector employees, including managers in the NHS, Le Grand (2006) found that public sector workers were generally more altruistic than their private sector counterparts; they wanted to provide a service to the public rather than focusing on financial performance or meeting organizational goals. Le Grand (2006) concludes that internationally, as well as in the UK, public service employees (including managers) 'report a greater concern for serving the community and helping others than private sector ones' so that 'it is hard to dispute the view that altruistic motivations are prevalent amongst the providers of public services'.

More specifically within the NHS, Wall (2001) conducted a tiny, in-depth, interview-based study of the careers of four top managers in the NHS, former national graduate trainees, recruited over a period of 30 years. These managers were not drawn into NHS management so much by a sense of vocation as by a sense of fascination and wanting to do something meaningful that made a difference. They had a long-term commitment to a public service ethos and to the localities and institutions in which they served. They were not much bothered about financial reward or formal external recognition; they wanted to engage in interesting, meaningful work on behalf of their fellow citizens.

In a later article, Wall (2004), a very experienced senior manager and management academic, advances the opinion that there are likely to be clashes between politically accountable managers trying to meet government targets and the clinicians with whom they work. And, in a survey article, Hunter (2002) characterizes the relationship between clinical professions, particularly doctors, and managers as one of tribal war, arguing that there continues to be a fundamental and presently irresolvable clash of values, aims and objectives between managers and doctors:

> Doctors insist upon treating individual patients in the manner they see to be in the patients' best interests and regard themselves as being accountable to the patients they serve and to their own conscience. In contrast, managers are concerned with the operation of the NHS as a whole and with ensuring that resources benefit the needs of a particular population or community rather than simply those of any single individual. (pp.67–68)

Hewison (2002) provides an ethnographic account of interviews with 26 middle managers in the NHS undertaken in 2000. Many of the managers interviewed had clinical backgrounds and so were 'hybrid managers', bringing with them professional values (not clearly defined) from practical patient care. Hewison found that clinicians who became managers assimilated many of the instrumental, rational values of management, e.g. a utilitarian concern for the future wellbeing of groups and wholes rather than individual needs within the resources allocated. However, hybrid and generic managers were likely to share a concern for meeting individual needs, and managers converged on the need to provide good services to patients. This finding is echoed in an Irish study about clinical versus managerial values (Carney 2006). Here it was found that, while there were differences between clinical and managerial values, and there was some distrust of each group for the values of the other, there was considerable convergence upon the need to provide good services for clients of health care. This kind of consensus allows cooperation.

Those detractors who want to see managers and management as the bringer of all ills to clinical health care will be dismayed by Hewison's finding that, 'The way some managers summarised the value base of their work would certainly not be out of place if expressed by a health professional' (Hewison 2002, p.562). This echoes Cox (1992, p.32): 'general managers have emphasized in interviews and displayed in observations an ability to show passionate concern for the values of care'.

If researchers like Cox, Hewison, Carney and Wall are to be believed, the actual behaviour and practice (as opposed to the espoused values) of managers may act as a vector for certain assumptions and practices that may impact negatively on professional values and concerns. However, this may well not be the intention of the managers themselves. Rather than seeing managers as the corrosive solvents of fundamental NHS values, they should be seen as part of the organization. If they ever did in fact espouse 'pure' private-sector management values, these continue to be considerably modified by the clinical and public sector values and practices with which they interact.

Managers are perhaps best seen in this context as pragmatic, functional chameleons. They are the bearers of certain beliefs and assumptions and the practitioners of certain habits that are bound up with organizing the successful use of resources to deliver services. The good that is sought as a result of management is determined by the context and organization in which management is practised. Thus in a public service, the good that is sought is likely to be the benefit of the public and it is to *that* end that management values and practices will be deflected. Within this ideological and institutional context, managers exert their pragmatic skills and aptitudes to deliver what the organization requires, often displaying great commitment to the 'product' (health care or other public service) to which the organization aspires.

WHAT DO CONTEMPORARY SENIOR NHS MANAGERS SAY ABOUT THEIR OWN VALUES?

To supplement the findings of the research literature, we decided to ask managers themselves what they believed their own values to be and how they felt that these might have changed. We focused on senior managers operating at executive level as Board or sub-Board members, principally within Primary Care Trusts, and including their provider-arm managers. These Trusts have responsibility for commissioning health care on behalf of their resident populations. At present, this can include devolved, semi-independent provision of community-based services. A further interview included Executive Team members from a Mental Health and Learning Disabilities provider background.

In 2008 we undertook group discussions with 27 Executive Team members working in the same Trusts in small groups. The participants came from a number of professional backgrounds. These included nursing (6), medical/public health (5) and physiotherapy (1). Six of these managers had worked in the commercial sector at some time. The majority had worked within the NHS for over 15 years, with 6 of them having 21–25 years' experience and 17 having between 26 and 41 years. The numbers of male and female managers were roughly even.

Semi-structured interviews/discussions took place in groups facilitated by one of the investigators, with a number of questions circulated prior to the meeting. However, at the meeting itself the discussion was allowed to evolve in the direction in which the teams took it. The provisional prompt questions were:

- What motivates you to come to work and do the job you are doing?

- What do you think are the values of NHS managers and how do you think they have changed in the last 10–15 years?

- Can you think of anything you did as a manager 10–15 years ago that you could not do now? What do you think this change points to about value changes?

- What is the one thing you would change about the NHS?

- Do you think your values are different from other professional groups within the NHS? How are they different?

- What do you think other professional groups view as your values? Are they right to hold this view?

- Where, if at all, do your views clash with those of other groups or national policy?

In addition, participants were encouraged to recall any incidents that they felt encapsulated the issues/values under discussion, i.e.:

- Can you recall an incident that illustrates what you are discussing?

One further question was added during some, but not all of the interviews, namely,

- Where do you think you learnt these values?

Meetings lasted between 40 minutes and one hour. Conversations were taped and reviewed by both investigators following the discussion. Participants also had the opportunity to submit comments confidentially following the meeting.

The main findings of the discussions can be summarized thematically.

BELIEVING IN THE MODEL OF THE NHS

Discussants displayed remarkable consistency and homogeneity in their commitment to basic values of the NHS. Unprompted, managers articulated a strong commitment to values that they identified as expressions of the NHS model. The most consistently cited were:

- focus on patients and improving their experience (both as groups and as individuals)
- maximizing health outcomes.

Commissioning managers went on to name equity, integrity and honesty as core values. Provider managers picked out values around seeking an evidence base, meeting targets, performance management and leadership.

Managers referred back to the NHS founding principles – universal care, free at the point of delivery, and spoke of 'believing in the model of the NHS'. There was talk of the vocational aspects of their commitment at the time when they entered the service.

CHANGING VALUES

There were different opinions across the service about whether values had changed. All of the service commissioner discussants felt that their own values had not changed significantly in recent years, although they did think that the value context within which they worked had changed considerably. The contextual changes raised concerned the introduction of political reforms. Some of the service provider managers believed values had changed, noting a greater and increasing impact from governmental reforms on their services over time.

THE DISTINCTIVENESS OF MANAGERIAL VALUES

Some managers did make reference to existing value statements, e.g. the IHM standards, the Nolan principles, nursing and medical codes. Managers did not see 'management values' as a distinct element within the NHS, although they did recognize that their role required a systematic approach to the provision of care that other professional roles might not require.

One Chief Executive commented upon the difficulty in identifying any single driving value, as the NHS is possibly a more complex organization than many commercial organizations (where the driving issue is primarily profit). He coined the phrase 'social profit' as a description of multiple outcomes that must be judged in total for their contribution to health and wellbeing. The issue of cost and the need to make hard decisions was recognized by the participants as integral to their work.

An interesting element of the discussions was the difficulty many discussants had in articulating individual values, the implication being that these were so obvious that they were rarely reflected upon. In addition, it was notable that values were easiest to express in terms of work goals. This would seem to support the view that managers' values have arisen from within the situation within which they work – that they are, indeed, 'pragmatic functionaries'.

A VERY DIFFERENT NHS IN FUTURE?

Managers expressed some identification with values associated with taking a systematic approach (which did not always benefit the individual patient), efficiency and economy. These were spoken of in ways that suggested they were intrinsic to their work. They showed more caution and distance when discussing issues such as competition and describing care as a commodity. The service providers in particular had seen the disadvantages of increased competitiveness and the decline of information-sharing in recent years. There were mixed views about the introduction of privatization. One Chief Executive commented that it would be 'a very different NHS in future'. Managers returned repeatedly to their central concern for patients and the vulnerability of many of the patient caseload. They supported the increased focus on improving the individual patient's experience, but were cautious about the implications of choice. Any benefits arising from the reforms were highlighted more often by the provider managers. It was recognized that there was now more respect for the patients and their individual rights.

Managers valued flexibility in their work and showed concern at perceived increased levels of centralization and arbitrary changes in policy. They also expressed a distance from the government level/ Department of Health operations and described incidents where they had been required to respond with little or no warning to central directives. There was generally little enthusiasm for further centrally driven, politically led, rapid organizational change and restructuring; this was seen as destabilizing. Managers did not see their purpose as defined by the reforms. They spoke of the tension and balance required to offset central concerns and local needs.

PART OF THE FAMILY

A fascinating element of the conversations arose as an aside in a number of discussions. Team members stated that where they had worked in organizations where they had felt their value set was not shared, then this had been (or could in future become) the cause of their move to another organization. However, one group felt that it was unusual to find managers who did not share their value set. Another group spoke of working in the NHS in previous years as being 'part of the family'. However, they also recognized the negative aspects of such an ethos – the potential for group pressure and condoning of inadequate service provision.

Managers' values were strongly held and deeply embedded. When asked where they had learned these values, the primary response was that they were learned from their parents and from managers with whom they worked. The commitment to an NHS vision of public service came through in a number of responses. One Director spoke of a short period in which she had worked in the private sector, but found that it 'felt really frivolous' so that she returned to the NHS. Another Director spoke of the NHS as 'the last bastion of the public sector'. Participants gave a sense of the importance they attached to their work and to the public nature of it. Working in the NHS was a life-long commitment.

RELATING TO HEALTH CARE PROFESSIONS AND OTHER GROUPS

Our discussants exhibited very little resentment of their fairly negative public image, seeming to accept its inevitability and to dismiss its significance. They appeared to draw strength from their common purpose and the importance that they themselves attributed to their work.

Managers rejected the notion that their values as a group were significantly different from those of other NHS professionals. However, they recognized that this was not always perceived by other professions, because of managers' role in controlling costs. One clinical manager spoke of the improved levels of real partnership and engagement, to which lip service had previously been paid. Another discussed how his dual roles as clinician and manager underlined the commonality of values held.

CONCLUSIONS

In line with previous studies we found that managers identified strongly with more altruistic values than those that might be expected from a commercially driven model of management. We were presented with a picture of articulate, committed senior managers who exhibited a strong sense of personal and group identity ranged round some central, common core values. Values did not appear to be often discussed, but implicit in all discussions was the confident assurance that the values expressed would be recognized and validated by the group. Managers saw their central values as patient-focused and as part of a long legacy of hospital management and public service as a whole. Provider managers had more sense that the value base was changing and showed greater acknowledgement of the language of the NHS reforms. However, there remained a sense of distance in all managers from elements of government reform language, particularly competition and perceived moves to privatization.

From this we infer that NHS managers have a strong value set. This focuses upon situational responses to being patient-centred and the practicalities of making a difference in health outcomes and equitable access. It is built upon a value base recognizable from the Nolan principles. On the whole, managers believed that their value base remained unchanged by recent changes within government philosophy. This was partly explained by differentiating personal and organizational values – it was felt that the organizational adjustment to recent health service changes was greater than any adjustment in personal beliefs. However, it was noticeable that the terminology used to describe personal and organizational beliefs was couched in language and ideas that have emerged within the NHS over the past 20 years – for example, the concern for healthier outcomes, the emphasis on equity and on patient focus. These elements of the NHS reforms appear to sit more comfortably with existing value sets and have been more easily integrated than ideas such as choice, competition and privatization, which have more potential room for conflict with ideas of equity, efficiency and teamwork as the managers understand it.

Management commitment to the NHS was life long. Between them, these managers had over 690 years of NHS service. The difficulties of the role are offset by the rewards of making a difference and seeing changes. The value set itself seems to act as a motivating force. Managers saw it as a common denominator in health care provision. As one said, 'At what point does someone become a manager with values rather than a nurse with values or a doctor with values?' Whilst they could perceive that other professions viewed them with suspicion and as lacking the values held by other groups, they felt this was not, in fact, the case.

These senior NHS managers seem to have a coherent, fairly conservative set of articulated values that are remarkably consistent across different groups and organizations and which reflect the founding values of the NHS. These values are held to be highly motivating and are oriented towards the practical end of improving health outcomes for patients and populations. Some consonant values have been added onto the core values that were held by NHS administrators before managers were introduced into the NHS in 1983. However, managers themselves believe that they can distinguish between personal values that are unchangeable and fundamental to their occupational role and identity and new, more epi-phenomenal values that have emerged from organizational change. In other words, despite their commitment to change and thinking about organizational culture, managers believe that there are things about themselves that cannot and will not change.

The commitment of managers to public service values and patients was impressive. However, we would like to end with a few critical comments and questions.

First, and most obviously, what managers articulate about their basic values may not be the most important aspect of values within their life and work. More research should be done actually to chart the relationship between articulated, espoused values and managers' values enacted in practice.

Second, while managers emphasize the similarity of their values with other professional groups in the NHS, and play down the significance of any perceived value differences and conflicts, there was some recognition that managers *are* perceived to be different in some ways (see Hunter 2002). In the context of increased teamworking alongside fragmentation of services, it is perhaps becoming increasingly important that managers should give more consideration to exploring and understanding value, and other differences, between groups. Without such understanding there may be unnecessary and misunderstood conflict. And, in this connection, it might perhaps be helpful if managers did more actively to articulate and exemplify their values to their clinical and lay colleagues and stakeholders, possibly through providing more exemplary case studies and stories of what their values mean and how they affect their work.

The discourse of the managers themselves showed that their values do change over time to respond to organizational and political change, despite their belief to the contrary. For two reasons it might be constructive for managers to be more conscious of the ways in which their values can be affected and change.

- First, because it is unrealistic to believe that individuals' values and identities are *not* changed in some ways by organizational and group norms; managers are no different to other individuals and groups in this regard.

- Second, because if managers are not able to recognize and work with their own changing values they may risk not being able to defend them and modify them consciously and voluntarily. This may endanger the long-term survival of the very values that managers claim most to care for. And if managers cannot critically, as well as comfortably, inhabit their own nuanced values then they may find themselves stuck with a rigid, inflexible identity that adapts poorly to change so that individuals are unable effectively to engage with it without breaking or withdrawing in the face of painful, cognitive and emotional dissonance. To put it strongly, if managers do not look to become more sophisticated exponents and critics of their occupational values, they may find that they are much more fragile and vulnerable than they currently hope they are.

To put all this much more positively, managers have a great deal to offer practically and theoretically in the field of values in health care. If they become more articulate, nuanced and interested in this area, and exemplify how values work with and for them, then they should be able to get into more interesting and complex discussions about health and care with their non-managerial colleagues and with the public. This should be empowering both for managers themselves in the face of political and other pressures and also for all those whose lives and work are affected by managerial influence. Managers, then, may need to become more curious and critical about their values. If they do this, they may find that they get on better with their colleagues (or at least know more about why they cannot get on with them) as well as with the public they rightly claim to serve and care for. This is not just about cosmetic spin so that managers are better understood and appreciated. It is also part of aspiring to be transparent and accountable to the citizenry upon whom the continuation of a publicly funded national health service depends.

RESPONSE
Moira Dumma

As a senior manager in the NHS for over 25 years, and one with a clinical background, there is much within this chapter that I recognize. In particular, the commitment of managers throughout the NHS to public service values and patient outcomes is something I come across often.

The authors report from the discussions with managers that they exhibited very little resentment of their fairly negative public image and a dismissal of its significance. I would argue this is not a view that is common at present. However, this is perhaps an issue where reactions vary according to circumstances. It is clear through recent experience in some parts of the NHS (where expectations of standards of care, patient safety, timeliness of service and achievement of targets have resulted in Chief Executives leaving posts) that there *is* a direct impact upon managers. In these situations the reports from other managers clearly reflect a concern about taking on these challenges in an unforgiving environment. Yet if we are to see changes that continually improve the patients' experience of services there must be accountability. The tension always remains for managers that being able to effect the change required means working with clinicians; but, as the authors point out, it also means that we managers have to become more curious and critical about our values.

The chapter does not refer to two significant areas for the NHS as we move forward and I believe that it is these two areas that offer the vehicles to do as the authors propose.

The Next Stage Review led by Lord Darzi[1] sets a very clear priority to increase clinical engagement – not only to ensure clinicians are encouraged into senior management posts but with an expressed objective from the Chief Executive of the NHS to see a clinician on every shortlist for Chief Executive posts. Yet it remains very difficult to attract clinicians to make that change. There are clearly a number of reasons for this and I highlight the two reported most frequently:

- first, the views of their peers that somehow they have 'gone over to the other side'

and

- second, because we do not articulate the role of management as the vehicle through which excellent care can be achieved.

The role of managers is to persuade clinicians that they can have as much, if not more, impact as a clinical leader on the community of patients and to demonstrate how that leadership can result in excellent care. We can only achieve this by being more transparent about, and discussing more broadly, the values by which we work, what they mean and how they affect our work.

The second area is the adoption of the NHS Constitution, which establishes the principles and values of the NHS in England, and formally documents the rights to which patients, public and staff are entitled, the pledges which the NHS is committed, and the responsibilities which the public, patients and staff owe to one another to ensure that the NHS operates fairly and effectively. Many, if not all, of these rights, responsibilities and pledges already existed, but the Constitution brings them together in one place for the first time.

The Constitution does not bestow any new rights to patients, public or staff, but draws together the principal existing rights under

---

1   The Darzi report: 'High quality care for all: NHS next stage review final report' (2008) was commissioned by the government and was presented to Parliament by the Secretary of State for Health. It was intended to create a vision for NHS care that would drive patient-choice-centred improvements in the quality of care over the next few decades.

law, and sets these out in a single document, balanced for the first time by responsibilities owed by patients, public and staff to one another. This articulation of the values of the NHS, which will be the duty of managers to ensure is enacted, does offer the framework upon which managers could do as the authors challenge. However, there is a real tension to be managed. As reported by the authors, if managers cannot see how their values align with the NHS Constitution and begin those complex discussions with clinicians, patients and others, it will be the very articulation of the values of the NHS that will challenge managers most.

REFERENCES

Carney, M. (2006) 'Positive and negative outcomes from values and beliefs held by health care clinician and non-clinician managers.' *Journal of Advanced Nursing 54*, 1, 111–119.

Clarke, J., Cochrane, A. and McLaughlin, E. (eds) (1994) *Managing Social Policy*. London: Sage.

Cox, D. (1992) 'Crisis and Opportunity in Health Service Management.' In R. Loveridge and K. Starkey (eds) *Continuity and Crisis in the NHS*. Milton Keynes: Open University Press.

Department of Health and Social Security (DHSS) (1983) *NHS Management Enquiry*. London: DHSS.

Department of Health (2002) *Code of Conduct for NHS Managers*. London: DoH.

Draper, H. (1998) 'Should Managers adopt the Medical Ethic? Reflections on Health Care Management.' In S. Dracopoulou (ed.) *Ethics and Values in Health Care Management*. London: Routledge.

Drucker, P. (1974) *Management: Tasks, Responsibilities, Practices*. Oxford: Butterworth-Heinemann.

du Gay, P. (ed.) (2005) *The Values of Bureaucracy*. Oxford: Oxford University Press.

Edwards, B. (1993) *The National Health Service: A Manager's Tale 1946–1992*. London: Nuffield Trust.

Ferlie, E., Ashburner, L., Fitzgerald, L. and Pettigrew, L. (1996) *The New Public Management in Action*. Oxford: Oxford University Press.

Hewison, A. (2002) 'Managerial values and rationality in the National Health Service.' *Public Management Review 4*, 4, 549–579.

Hunter, D. (2002) 'A Tale of Two Tribes: The Tension between Managerial and Professional Values.' In B. New and J. Neuberger (eds) *Hidden Assets: Values and Decision Making in the NHS*. London: King's Fund.

Institute of Healthcare Management (IHM) (2001) 'IHM Healthcare Management Code.' London: IHM.

Lawton, A. (1998) *Ethical Management for the Public Services*. Buckingham: Open University Press.

Le Grand, J. (2006) *Motivation, Agency, and Public Policy*. Oxford: Oxford University Press.

Locke, R. (1996) *The Collapse of the American Management Mystique*. Oxford: Oxford University Press.

Pattison, S. (1997) *The Faith of the Managers: When Management Becomes Religion*. London: Cassell.

Pollitt, C. (1993) *Managerialism in the Public Sector* (2nd edn). Oxford: Basil Blackwell.

Pugh, D. and Hickson, D. (1989) *Writers on Organizations* (4th edn). London: Penguin Books.

Ranson, S. and Stewart, J. (1994) *Management for the Public Domain: Enabling the Learning Society*. Basingstoke: Macmillan.

Strong, P. and Robinson, J. (1990) *The NHS under New Management*. Milton Keynes: Open University Press.

Wall, A. (2001) *Being a Health Service Manager – Expectations and Experience: A Study of Four Generations of Managers in the NHS*. London: The Nuffield Trust.

Wall, A. (2004) 'Is Health Service Management a Profession?' In S. Pattison and R. Pill (eds) *Values in Professional Practice*. Oxford: Radcliffe.

Chapter 11

Health Care Professions and their Changing Values: Pulling Professions Together

Huw Thomas and Stephen Pattison

INTRODUCTION

Aneurin Bevan, the minister in charge of founding the National Health Service (NHS) in the late 1940s, made no mention of professional, organizational or personal values as an important constituent part of providing effective health care. Rather, he talked in general terms of the importance of alleviating anxiety about finance and payment in times of sickness, leaving the adumbration of more detailed values and principles to others (Klein 2007).

Sixty years after the founding of what is often taken to be one of the main vehicles and expressions of fundamental British social *mores*, the NHS is filled with values talk. The overt invocation and expression of values has arisen in the context of huge social and organizational change; in particular, it has coincided with the rise of the market society and ideas of market and consumerism in public service. This is not surprising, given the origin of 'value' in market and economic relationships (Pattison 2004). Where politics and morality cede space to a rhetoric of technique, organization and management, it seems that the language of values enters to fill – or even perhaps to disguise – a fundamental void around conflicting ends, purposes and functions. In the face of enormous diversity, pluriformity and complexity, talk of values has become one of the main ways in which professionals, their employers and the public can discourse on issues of identity, purpose, expectation and the common good.

At the time of writing (summer 2009), it looks as if the era of the market society and market thinking may be coming to an end in the face of recession and economic crisis. This is likely to require a reorientation in public services, not least because funding is likely to become much scarcer. In this context, it will be interesting to see whether values talk survives as a main means for groups and individuals to discuss their direction, goals and function. Perhaps the languages of religion, ethics, or political debate and dissent will reassert themselves in a world where fundamental decisions have to be made about social cohesion, conflict and value (Sandel 2009).

Be that as it may, it is clear that there will always have to be some discussion and vocabulary for articulation that allows individuals, professionals, professions and organizations to talk to, and with, each other about roles, ideals and expectations. If professionals, users and institutions are to pull together with some commonality of goal, intent, ends and means, then, in one form or another, they will have to engage within the field of values, whether this is done implicitly or explicitly. Failure to do this is likely to result in a frustrating dissipation of energy and good will as people work against, rather than with, each other.

Whether the explicit language of values continues to be of significance in personal, professional and organizational life cannot be determined at present. At this point, our purpose is to take stock of the insights that have emerged about changing professional values, and values talk, during the course of producing this book. Here in this final chapter, then, we reflect on some significant themes and understandings. We then draw out some practical and theoretical implications for those involved in the NHS and its future (including its users) before setting out an agenda for research and enquiry. We conclude with some thoughts about the future of the professions in the NHS.

MAIN INSIGHTS AND THEMES
Diversity and variability of discourses and contexts
One prominent theme to have emerged from the essays in this book is that there is a great diversity of ways in which values and talk of values are, and have been, used in professional life in the NHS. Most obvious, perhaps, are the differences in the public discourses of particular

professions. Mental health nursing is a prime example of an occupation that has reflected on its role in an increasingly value-related way for some time. In the field of genetic counselling, too, values are central to important discussions. The vulnerability of the users of these services, and the intimate contact that professionals have with them, press these kinds of concerns into the consciousness of professional institutes and individual professionals. Broader changes in social *mores* are important, too; mental health, for example, has for some decades been a focus of those generally sceptical about the medicalization of Western life.

Yet, to some extent all users of health care are vulnerable, and health care is necessarily an intimate matter. So it is interesting that in a profession like pharmacy the discussion of values and ethics is relatively recent and, we might venture, slightly underdeveloped. Why might this be? The concerns and pressures of community pharmacy are clearly very different from those encountered by industrial pharmacists, for example, and perhaps this has inhibited the development of a public discourse in relation to values and ethics in the profession. Most professions include people in a variety of settings, and reflections on values may not have the same salience in each. Moreover, different settings may engender and support very different perspectives on what constitute important values for that particular occupational situation. For example, professionals who work in settings that have long been commercial – such as community pharmacy – will tend to have systematically different evaluations of the ethical significance of markets in health care from professionals in settings with no such history, like nursing. The case studies included in this book show the way in which trends in the NHS are creating fragmentation in some professions (e.g. GPs, and, possibly, hospital chaplains). It remains to be seen how these may complicate their public discussions about values.

Professional identity and context

The case studies also underline the ways values are implicated in the formation or consolidation of professional identity. Freidson's (2001) suggestion that different professions may still claim to pursue distinctive transcendent values does not appear to translate easily into the lived reality of professional lives and discourses. The process is actually messy and unresolved; it occurs at many levels and in various settings. The accounts of general medical practice, mental health nursing and chaplaincy explore this at an institutional and collective level. In each case, there has been collective and (to varying degrees) public discussion about what it is that distinguishes the profession in terms of its value-base, not just in its skills and expertise. The settings for this are varied.

As the examples of mental health nursing and general practice illustrate, public enquiries, often governmentally sponsored, are important *fora* in which arguments over values are rehearsed. Important, too, are workplaces – such as those in which unionization has been discussed by hospital chaplains. The *setting* has implications for who can be involved in the discussion. As Hannigan points out, even government-sponsored enquiries can impose quite severe restrictions on who has an input into a discussion. Debate within a professional institute tends to be even more restricted; as are the aforementioned workplace discussions.

Roles, modes and judgements

A view of the appropriate role and mode of working of a profession will inevitably include a view (and an embedded evaluation) of the significance of other professions and service users. Thus, a view about whose judgements should influence decisions in relation to a particular health care episode will involve evaluations of the competence, and significance (including the moral significance) of the various actors involved in the episode. This is clearly shown in some of the case studies in this book: the training doctor in Monrouxe and Sweeney's account of medical education attaches no significance to the trainee doctor's opinions but also – implicitly – no significance to his (the trainee's) conscience. In genetic counselling, we see counsellors struggling with the weight to be put on the welfare of various parties who will be influenced by the matter at hand, and also on the weight to be attached to their own judgements as professional counsellors.

In Chapter 2, Edgar reviews the various roles that patients have been expected to play in the NHS since its inception. His review draws largely on official discourses, and hence espoused values, about patient/professional relations. There are clear evaluations built into ideas such as those that a patient should be a largely passive recipient of professional advice or a consumer of health care 'products'. These include judgements about what the patient is capable of, and what the patient should be encouraged to become capable of. They also involve judgements about what constitutes a good life for the patient, and who is best able to judge what constitutes a good life. Such judgements, and the social interactions through which they are played out, are embedded in wider social relations; health professionals, patients (and friends and families) interact as embodied entities. As such, they are gendered, class-located, of a certain age, and so on. Sayer (2005) argues persuasively that these attributions come freighted with evaluations. In real-life encounters, therefore, between professionals and between professionals and patients, the role that values play will be impossible to comprehend fully without placing the actors in their wider social context.

Values, organizations and politics

While chapters in this book have provided some material for readers who wish to think about professional/patient interaction at a personal level, they have done less to pursue ways in which patients and professionals might relate to more strategic issues about health care. Hannigan's account of public enquiries into mental health demonstrates that, historically, the public has not been expected to play much of a role in these kinds of strategic overviews. But, overall, the book does little to follow up Edgar's discussion of whether and how value commitments of health care users should be incorporated into discussions about the big issues facing the NHS. A well-established approach to addressing this issue is representative democracy – for example, with MPs (through Parliament) expressing the values of the wider public. In relation to health care this has the same strength (simplicity) and obvious limitations (lack of citizen engagement, complexity of representing the values of a diverse, even fractured, society) as contemporary representative democracy in general. As Edgar points out in his chapter, attempts to engage the wider public in informed discussions of strategic choices in health care have tended to fail.

The second approach (which follows one interpretation of what it is to be consumer/patient focused) polls users and potential users about their views and priorities. In this approach, the user is reactive, largely passive and, typically, uninformed about all but her or his personal experience. This approach to tapping in to user views in effect encourages users to be self-interested and insular; in that respect it exemplifies a clear, and contestable, value-commitment. In addition, it does very little directly to encourage health care users to reflect upon their values or deepen their understanding of their own values, and values in general. In a society where there is an increasingly crude approach to thinking about values and about public life (Fevre 2000), this approach will tend to increase the sense of alienation felt by professionals who wish to develop a practice that is consistent with a sophisticated, historically grounded value-orientation, as Sellman tries to do in relation to nursing.

Perhaps the most restrictive setting of all in terms of who has an input into influencing what are considered to be appropriate values in health care is the one-to-one training of the novice professional by the experienced practitioner. Monrouxe and Sweeney analyse the role of values in the professional socialization of individual doctors. Their data captures the intensity of the experience in which student doctors attempt to reconcile their own view of patients and how they might be treated with that of their instructor. As Hurwitz points out, the power relations at work in the episode are significant. They make it overwhelmingly likely that in the short term at least there will be just one outcome: somehow or other, the lone novice will find a way of adjusting and reconciling his (in this case) values with what his instructor has done – and which he, the novice, will presumably be expected to do in future. The values of patients, Hurwitz notes, play no part in this process. Whether this value congruence 'sticks' is, of course, another matter. As Pill points out, the values we hold are affected by our experience of life, including the circumstances in which we work, while Hoggett, Mayo and Miller (2009) emphasize the significance of personal biography in the development of value orientations among professionals. It would be fascinating to do a longitudinal qualitative study of a large cohort of health care professionals to get some kind of insight into the nature of these changes and reasons for them.

Overt discussion of values

One startling aspect of the episodes Monrouxe and Sweeney describe is the apparent absence of overt discussion of values by the protagonists. Values are central to what they are engaged in, but are largely unspoken, and invisible. Something similar appears to be the case among NHS managers. Pattison and McKeown make the point that their interviewees appear to be lacking practice in discussing values overtly. Sarangi refers to value-inflected discussions about appropriate orientations among academic writers on genetic counselling, but his case study of the practice of counselling appears to show a marked lack of reflection on the part of counsellors on the implications of their style and approach to counselling. With the exceptions of mental health nurses and hospital chaplains there is little evidence that the health care professions reviewed here have an established practice of widespread and sustained discussion of values. Why might this be? Perhaps some of the following reasons might severally or together help to account for this strange silence:

- The hierarchies within and between health professions inhibit discussion of values. As in the case of the novice doctor, people are pretty much dragooned into at least acting according to a certain set of values, whatever their personal reservations.

- Professionals mostly lack the skill, confidence or vocabulary to engage in discussions about values. In a society where deep political or religious commitment is relatively rare, and generally regarded as a private matter, most people are ill-equipped to engage in sustained discussion of value issues.

- There are no obvious vehicles or *fora* for such discussions – particularly across professional boundaries.

- Values are regarded as either self-evident or epi-phenomenal. So they are not worth discussing because they are taken either to be unchangeable and eternal, or to sit above everyday life and practice in such a way that they do not really influence it. Values talk, then, is basically redundant chatter.

Yet, as Sayer (2005) points out, beliefs about what matters (whether such beliefs are labelled as 'moral' or as being about 'values') are one of the bases for critiques of how social life is organized. Sellman's chapter on general adult nursing, and Hockley's response to it, provide ample evidence of this phenomenon in relation to a changing NHS. It is values deemed central to, indeed constitutive of, nursing that are used to justify resistance by nurses to changes in the way they are expected to work. Again, Chapter 10 shows managers appearing to justify what they are doing (which has involved introducing changes bitterly resented by some other professions) as being consistent with established values underpinning the NHS. Edgar's analysis in Chapter 2 might induce some scepticism as to the historical accuracy of that claim; perhaps the espoused values of managers are at variance with the values they enact.

But their very talking in this way may well illustrate the way in which values are used to justify change and attempt to create a coalition of support for it.

When people use values to justify opposition to some aspect of their working conditions, in part they will do so because they wish to align personal values with those shaping their working lives. One need not accept MacIntyre's philosophical framework to agree with Sellman that the necessary institutionalizing of care affects the nature of what it is that is offered. In such cases, there are difficult personal judgements to be made by sensitive professionals about whether the changes matter enough to wish to change the institution. Complete congruence of personal values with institutional values is unlikely. Indeed, if one thinks of the NHS as an institutional vehicle for supporting many kinds of (professional) practices of caring, then the possibility that all professionals can find themselves in harmony with the value environment in which they work is remote. It is all the more important, therefore, that professionals become accustomed to open, sustained discussions about values in relation to their work.

Interprofessional working

Provision for, and development of, meaningful interprofessional dialogue is vital if Freidson's (2001) recommendation of supporting greater professional authority in the face of bureaucratic and market mechanisms and values is to be taken seriously (see Pill and Hannigan, Chapter 1). If this is to happen, there must be some way of reconciling the inevitable overlap of concerns, and differences of outlook and values, of the plethora of professions that now exist in the NHS. Historically, this reconciliation has been achieved by an occupational hierarchy that has imposed the concerns and values of doctors (and, on occasion, those of certain specialisms within their ranks) on all other professions in health care. Even a brief experience of an NHS acute hospital shows that in this important setting for health care the hierarchy is in some ways unchanged at the operational level, whatever changes managerial intervention has wrought more generally. The necessity perceived by chaplains to become professionalized in a rather specific sense if they are to be a *bona fide* part of the health care team illustrates in a different way the way in which occupations can only address their marginality in health care on terms dictated by other professions.

Interprofessional dynamics and power relations cannot be divorced from the way that values are conceived and discussed (Sayer 2005). A call for generalized 'professional autonomy' (in certain spheres) can only be given credence in a complex organizational setting if there is an explicit acknowledgement that this is, in effect, a call for a certain kind of power relation within the organization and that this arrangement will both instantiate and promote certain sets of values. Again, this needs to be acknowledged and discussed openly by all likely to be directly affected.

Implications for practitioners

This book's major practical implication is that practitioners need to be aware of, sensitive to, and articulate about, values – both their own, and those of others. Without understanding the role that personal and organizational values play in a complex and dynamic context, professional effectiveness is likely to be heavily compromised. Achieving an understanding is not always easy.

The book's historical perspective underlines the dynamic, changing nature of value commitments. To be sure, values are not things that are changed at the drop of a hat, but, over time, individuals and organizations (including professional institutes) often do amend and adjust their sets of values. Such changes typically arise in response to circumstances in work (at the individual level, the socialization of professionals is an example). At other times, it is changes in the context of professionals' work that are important. Changes in social thought and *mores* in the 1960s and 1970s, for example, fundamentally affected mental health nursing. But the kinds of responses will differ from one profession to another, because each has a different history and is situated differently in the web of social and power relations that constitute the NHS. So, for example, the notion of patient-centredness promoted in the NHS plays itself out very differently in different kinds of professional work. The case studies of Monrouxe and Sweeney, Sarangi, and Swift show three very different orientations of the professional to the patient, each incorporating different sets of power relations. As Edgar points out in Chapter 2, at other times again, patient-centredness has acquired primarily a consumerist meaning. Sometimes, values become more entrenched (rather than modified) in the face of change, as part of the process of resistance – in the case of adult general nursing, this is what appears to be happening in some settings.

Health care is a multi-professional task, and those involved – especially those managing the process – need to be sensitive to the scope for value-shift and potential congruence in values, and the possibility of there being a 'digging in' over value commitments. Judging what may happen, and its significance, is never easy. At the very least, it involves engaging with fellow professionals as people with value-commitments rather than simply fellow 'cogs' in a giant machine. This can, but need not always, mean explicitly talking about values. Careful attention to how work is done, for example, is just one way of beginning to understand the values of professionals involved.

This sensitivity to all those involved in health care (including users of services) as people with serious value commitments is more important than it has ever been because of the increasing heterogeneity of professionals and service-users. Some professions, and still more specialisms within them, remain heavily gendered and class-biased, but overall the composition of the health care professions has become more socially diverse (even in chaplaincy). And, of course, users of NHS services are more diverse, and often conscious of it.

In these circumstances, easy or lazy assumptions about how people see things, and what they value, should be avoided. Swift, in his response to the chapter on chaplaincy, provides an instructive case study of what this kind of sensitivity can mean when someone dies in hospital. It is clear that making assumptions about shared ethico-religious frameworks is perilous for professionals and service-users, but this need not create tensions or undue anxiety because people understand when others respect the fact that individuals' values are to be respected, even if they do not always understand what those values are. Genuine attempts to find out what matters to people will rarely be rebuffed. On the other hand, a failure to appreciate and engage with what matters to others is unlikely to facilitate creative and responsive relationships.

AN AGENDA FOR RESEARCH AND ENQUIRY

Given the prevalence and apparent importance of values and values talk in health care, it is surprising that the area has not been more thoroughly researched and explored. Values talk seems largely to be seen as above or beneath the curiosity of researchers into the NHS. However, the variety of research methods deployed in this book shows not only that values can be explored, and unearthed, in many ways, but also that there is a considerable agenda for further exploration. It is only possible to provide a selection of areas and directions for investigation here.

In the Introduction to this book we set out five ways in which we thought references to values might be involved in the changing NHS. They were:

1. legitimizing action and organizational arrangements

2. helping to coordinate action

3. disciplining and helping to manage people

4. justifying change and resistance to change

5. helping to create and consolidate identity.

If these categories are taken as hypotheses, or even informed speculations, the evidence and discussions of this book – including those earlier in this chapter – have mostly had a bearing on numbers 1, 4 and 5. They have not addressed 2 and 3. We will deal with the prospects and opportunities for potential further research using headings derived from these points.

Legitimizing action and organizational arrangements

The case studies provide examples of values being used both to justify and resist organizational arrangements – current, and aspirational. When backs are against the wall – as Sellman and Hockley suggest adult general nurses may often feel – then core values are used as points of reference in thinking through how things could, and should, be done better. But how do values, and reflections on values, bear on the more mundane day-to-day practice of health care? The evidence of interviews with a small group of managers (Chapter 10) is that little reflection on values takes place day to day. It would be useful to know how common this is, and to what extent there might be 'value drift' among health care professionals if they have no time or incentive (or perhaps practice) in reflecting on values. Do they unwittingly, perhaps subtly, shift their value commitments? If so, what are the causes of this phenomenon? And what impact does it have, both consciously and unconsciously, on the professionals in question?

Closely related to this is the question of the significance of a culture of targets for the kinds of values professionals espouse and enact. In Sellman's chapter on nursing, and Hockley's response, the target culture is castigated for its potentially corrosive effects on the values of adult nursing; it also features in Pill's chapter on general practice. But it does not feature so prominently in other chapters. This may be a consequence of the particular lenses and data used in those chapters, but it may also reflect the different situations in which different professionals find themselves. The interviews with NHS managers suggest that at the very least values inimical to a crude focus on measurable outcomes remain important. The relationships between targets, cultures and values need far more investigation.

Ethnographic research projects that examine the day-to-day reality of life in the NHS would be one way of addressing these kinds of questions. Such projects could also shed some light on how the values of service users might influence the way they use and act within the NHS. Hoggett *et al.*'s (2009, p.7) research involving 'extended contact' with 30 development workers over a period of 18 months provides an alternative quasi-ethnographic approach that has delivered interesting findings about personal ethical dilemmas among professionals.

Helping to coordinate action

The case studies in this book shed little light on the way in which values may be involved in interprofessional working. Given that interprofessional teamwork and fluid professional responsibilities are being encouraged within the NHS (see Chapters 1 and 2), there is a big gap in research here. An important aspect of this part of the research agenda must be to question whether values used to help disparate groups work together can ever be anything other than platitudes of the kind found in the recent NHS Constitution. What might a more sophisticated or subtle value-base for health care look like? If it requires a notion of human flourishing, for example (as might seem plausible), can a notion non-contestable enough to be usable be arrived at in a multi-faith, multi-cultural context that can help not only with prioritizing fractures and sprains, but also guide discussion of interventions in fertility, gene therapy and other radical action. Users/patients are allegedly 'partners' too, and there remains an enormous gap in knowledge about the way in which the values of users are, and could be, inserted into the complex ongoing negotiations that characterize health care in practice. In respect to this, Swift's account of a funeral of a patient, referred to earlier in this chapter, gestures towards a large and important area of investigation.

More generally, the book does not look at what happens when values of two professions clash – an important and long-neglected topic. For example, what relationship, if any, might there be between apparent resentment on the part of some professions of the power and authority of doctors (and their distinctive perspectives of patients and their needs) over some aspects of health care (as evidenced by anecdotal evidence, at least) and interprofessional organizational politics that involve struggles over the redistribution of some health care roles?

The role of values in managing and disciplining professionals

Almost all professional codes are based on some kind of vision of fundamental values and principles. Codes and values are then applied to individual practitioners, often in disciplinary contexts. Values are also important in helping professionals to remain motivated and committed to their work, finding expression perhaps in the slightly old-fashioned sounding notion that professional work is in some way vocational and requires more from its practitioners than simply blind conformity to a set of predetermined practices and rules. It would be highly desirable to see notions like vocation and discipline more thoroughly explored by researchers so that something more of the complexity of the interaction between values and actual occupational labour might become visible.

Justifying change and resistance to change

As noted several times already in this chapter, values are fundamental both to justifying and resisting change. It would be good to see researchers paying more attention to the kinds of values that are used in these ways by different professions and in different contexts. Are there some kinds of values that are likely to be more persuasive or compelling within particular settings or organizations? Are these most likely to be distinctively professional values based on claims to particular knowledge and expertise? Or is it more likely that appeals to overall communal goods, such as closeness to and respect for the patient, are likely to be more compelling in the public arena? Again, it would be desirable to become a great deal clearer about the nature and types of discourse that are used by different groups for different purposes in different contexts as these can vary enormously. There are opportunities here not only for sociologists and discourse analysts, but also for ethicists and rhetoricians to cast light on discussions that otherwise pass without much overt analysis.

Helping to create and consolidate identity

A major theme of this book is the recognition that values are intrinsically bound up with complex discussions and manoeuvres about group and professional identity. To have a particular professional identity is, in many ways to have a particular set of espoused, if not enacted, values that differentiates one professional group and set of skills from another. Given the drive towards the breakdown of professional exclusivity in the interests of providing seamless and flexible service to NHS users, it would seem important to understand better the dynamics of professional identity formation and consolidation, both sociologically and philosophically. This might enable what might seem like trivial turf wars in practice to be seen in a new and more constructive light. It is impossible to conceive of a world in which health care workers will be able to merge their values completely into one vast, generic identity because a sense of history, location, expertise and belonging are important components of fulfilling work. However, it is important to understand better the forces that maintain and influence values and identity and how this is worked out between and within groups. Observational ethnography might be one important method to apply here so that justice can be done to the internal discussion and meaning-making that goes on in professions and professionals, both intra-professionally and within wider social and institutional contexts.

THE FUTURE OF PROFESSIONS IN THE NHS

Professions and their values do not exist in a bubble, nor are they unchanging. A dynamic relationship exists between individual professionals, their occupational groups, the institutions in which they work, and the society in which those institutions are situated. At any point in time, intra-, inter- and extra-professional contextual factors bear upon professional self-understanding and practice.

Despite the critique of professions and professionals that has been advanced over the past 50 years, and despite the public's expressed anxiety and sometimes contempt for those who appear to set themselves up as experts while in fact displaying arrogance and incompetence in practice, there is no real appetite to denigrate the knowledge and usefulness of health care practitioners. While service-users might report unfortunate experiences, poor manners and inadequate practice on the part of some of those professionals they encounter in health care, the NHS remains one of Britain's most popular institutions – officially beloved by both left- and right-wing politicians as the treasured expression of the most fundamental national values. At the heart of the NHS lies the provision of professionally led and informed service. So there seems no prospect that professions and professionals will cease to exist.

There is, however, every prospect that health care organizations, professions and professionals will continue to have to change radically both their practices and the ways in which they think about themselves, individually and corporately. Identity and values are not fixed, even if part of the ways in which people tend to think about these categories tends to be one of reifying them a-historically so that they appear to be unchanging and eternally valid. Freidson (2001) argues that professions and professionalism will continue to be important because they allow particular kinds of specialized knowledge and expertise that are of use to society at large to continue to develop. A profession serves as a kind of hot house for the nurturance and preservation of particular kinds of necessary knowledge. However, he does helpfully recognize that professional claims to be left alone to develop on their own and 'do their own thing' are unlikely completely to be accepted within late capitalist society. Professions are hemmed in by, on the one side, those marketers who require them to provide their riches more economically, efficiently and in a more customer-focused way, and on the other, by those bureaucrats who require of them greater consistency and accountability to those who employ or pay for them. Bureaucratic, economic and professional values are in conflict to some extent.

It is very unlikely that this conflict will cease; indeed, it is likely to become more intense in the NHS over the next few years as resources dwindle while politicians, managers and economists respectively seek to curb professional autonomy and power, simultaneously requiring more flexible working and lower wages. In this context, the future of professions and professionals is likely to become ever more turbulent and to change more, and more quickly. It is at moments like this that values talk might become much more important as individuals and groups negotiate for influence, power and relative autonomy. But this will be against a background in which most professionals have already recognized that they will never have complete individual or intra-professional autonomy ever again. The days of the single-handed, autonomous practitioner who occupied the same position and did the same tasks with the same people for 30 or 40 years are over.

The changes we have observed in this volume are likely to accelerate and to become more challenging as the years go on. And with these, there will be fundamental challenges to professional work, identity and values. It is to be hoped that a volume such as this will at least throw some sideways light on the forces and ideas that might be relevant to these challenges, so that individual professionals, their professions, the organizations in which they work and the people they serve can meet a difficult future to some extent forewarned and forearmed. The individual, organizational and social costs of failing to recognize the importance of values in sustaining and guiding the motivation and provision of professional health care could be enormous. So our hope is that this book will serve as a starting point for a much wider, more articulate and more serious consideration of the relation of values to professions and health care.

REFERENCES

Fevre, R. (2000) *The Demoralization of Western Culture: Social Theory and the Dilemmas of Modern Living.* London: Continuum.

Freidson, E. (2001) *Professionalism: The Third Logic.* Cambridge: Polity.

Hoggett, P., Mayo, M. and Miller, C. (2009) *The Dilemmas of Development Work. Ethical Challenges in Regeneration.* Bristol: Policy Press.

Klein, R. (2007) 'Values Talk in the (English) NHS.' In S. Greer and D. Rowland (eds) *Devolving Policy, Diverging Values: The Values of the United Kingdom's National Health Services.* London: The Nuffield Trust.

Pattison, S. (2004) 'Understanding Values.' In S. Pattison and R. Pill (eds) *Values in Professional Practice: Lessons for Health, Social Care and Other Professionals.* Oxford: Radcliffe.

Sandel, M. (2009) *Markets and Morals.* The Reith Lectures 2009. London: BBC.

Sayer, A. (2005) *The Moral Significance of Class.* Cambridge: Cambridge University Press.

List of Contributors

David Badcott is an honorary research fellow in the Centre for Applied Ethics at Cardiff University, and a retired pharmacist.

Paul Ballard is professor emeritus in the Cardiff School of Religious and Theological Studies.

Bronwen Davies is a mental health nurse and team leader of the North Cardiff Crisis Resolution and Home Treatment Team.

Moira Dumma is an occupational therapist, and chief executive of South Birmingham Primary Care Trust.

Andrew Edgar is a senior lecturer in philosophy at Cardiff University.

Ben Hannigan is a senior lecturer in the Cardiff School of Nursing and Midwifery Studies, Cardiff University.

Christine Hockley is a sister/emergency nurse practitioner in Bristol, and a senior lecturer in nursing at the University of the West of England.

Brian Hurwitz is a general practitioner and also D'Oyly Carte professor of medicine and the arts at King's College London.

Julia McKeown is a health care manager and director of Fulcrum JRC Limited.

Lynn Monrouxe is a senior lecturer in medical education and director of medical education research at the Cardiff School of Medicine, Cardiff University.

Alan Nathan is a pharmacist and also visiting lecturer in the Department of Pharmacy at King's College London.

Roisin Pill is professor emerita at the Cardiff School of Medicine, and an honorary fellow of the Royal College of General Practitioners.

Stephen Pattison is professor of religion, ethics and practice at Birmingham University, and a member of the ethics committee of the Royal College of General Practitioners.

Srikant Sarangi is professor in language and communication, and director of the Health Communication Research Centre at Cardiff University.

Derek Sellman is a principal lecturer in the Faculty of Health and Life Sciences at the University of the West of England.

Heather Skirton is a genetic counsellor and professor in applied health genetics at Plymouth University.

Kieran Sweeney is a general practitioner and also a senior lecturer in General practice at the Peninsula Medical School at the Universities of Exeter and Plymouth.

Chris Swift is lead chaplain at the Leeds Teaching Hospitals NHS Trust.

Huw Thomas is a reader in the Cardiff School of City and Regional Planning, Cardiff University.

Paquita de Zulueta is a general practitioner, and honorary senior lecturer in General practice at Imperial College London.

Subject Index

Author Index